VET VIEW

For Vet-Job Aspirants

VET VIEW

For Vet-Job Aspirants

Dr. Samik Kumar Paul

2025

Astral Cracker

A Division of

Astral International Pvt. Ltd.

New Delhi – 110 002

ISBN: 978-93-5919-953-5

Published by : **Astral Cracker**
A Division of
Astral International Pvt. Ltd.
– ISO 9001:2015 Certified Company –
4736/23, Ground Floor, Ansari Road,
Darya Ganj, New Delhi-110 002
Ph. 011-43549197, 23278134
e-mail: info@astralint.com
Website: www.astralint.com

Printed at : **Replika Press**

Acknowledgement

At first I would like to express my deepest sense of unbound gratitude and indebtedness to my perspicacious reverend sir, Prof. Purnendu Biswas, Ex-Vice Chancellor, West Bengal University of Animal and Fishery Sciences for his overall guidance during writing and contribution for this book. His whole hearted support and constructive criticism acted as a source of inspiration for proper writing of this book.

I feel immense pleasure to express my heartiest thanks to Dr. Yograj Tamang, Director of Animal Husbandry and Veterinary Service, West Bengal and Prof. Nilotpal Ghosh, Dean, F/O VAS, W.B.U.A.F.S for their valuable suggestion without which this book would not have become a reality.

I take this opportunity to express my deepest sense of indebtedness and gratitude to Dr. Shuvendu Halder, Assistant Director, ARD for his instinct guidance, keen interest, foresight, continuous encouragement and expert suggestions during writing of this book. It was his inspiration and invaluable motivation with which the journey was started for writing this book. I am sincerely obliged and grateful to him.

I would like to express my sincere gratitude and acknowledgement to Dr. Gurucharan Datta, Vice President IVA and member VCI, for his inspiration, necessary advice and active help during preparation of this book.

I would like to convey my sincere regards to Dr. Sujoy Sikder, WBCS (Exe), Dr. Sumanta Roy, WBCS (EXE), Dr. Jyotirmay Chanda, BLDO and Dr. Chandrachur Raha, AD, ARD who have inspired me continuously to write this book.

I am sincerely obliged and thankful to all the authors and contributors, Dr. Prabhakar Biswas, Dr. Arun Mondal, Dr. Sougat Chakrabarty, Dr. Tapan Sadhukhan, Dr. Ratanti Sarkhel, Dr. Sourav Maiti, Dr. Abhijit Nandi, Dr. Kinshuk Maity, for their valuable contributions for this book. My sincere gratitude goes to them who contributed their time and expertise to this book.

I also like to extend my deepest sense of gratitude to Dr. Ziaul Hassan, Dr. Satyendranath Das, Dr. Susanta Kumar Manna, Dr. Tarani Kanta Bera, Dr. Debrup Roy, Dr. Rudraprasad Sengupta for helping me in the process of proof checking and editing.

It will be a serious injustice in my part if I shall not acknowledge and express my heartiest gratitude to my beloved classmates, Dr. Ziaul Hassan, Dr. Shib Sankar Saren, Dr. Shiba Prasad Patra, IPS, Dr. Sudipta Santra,WBCS(Exe),Dr. Bulbul Bakchi,WBCS(Exe), Dr. Satyabrata Halder, WBCS(Exe) for their whole-hearted co-operation rendered through out the writing of this book.

I wish to offer my heartiest thanks to my beloved juniors and senior Dr. Hemanta Kr Das, Dr. Ambika Prasad Mishra, Dr. Ajgar Ali Mondal, Dr. Nayan Bantul, Dr. Sayantan Raj, Dr. Susmita Pal, Dr. Priyanka Sarkar, Dr. Tapas Kundu, Dr. Koushik Pal, Dr. Biswadip Rakshit, Dr. Samim Reja for their constant inspiration and encouragement as well as friendly assistance throughout the writing of this book.

I bestow my sincere gratitude to Astral International Pvt. Ltd for enabling me to publish this book.

No formal word is sufficient to convey my heartiest thanks to my beloved wife Dr. Devapriya Har, my son Rishik, my mother and rest of my family who supported and encouraged me in spite of all the time it took me away from them.

Last but not least, I humbly ask for forgiveness from everyone who has supported me over the years but whose names I have omitted.

With sincere appreciation and regards.

Dr. Samik Kumar Paul

Preface

The book "Vet View: For Vet-Job Aspirants" has been prepared for the students/ candidates who are preparing for various competitive examination at the state and national level in the field of Animal Husbandry and Veterinary Science, specifically for appearing various job interview. Often in related interview in different State PSC or in national level examination students find difficulty to collect and cover study material for all the disciplines to prepare themselves for said examination and fails to crack these milestone. This model book catering the needs of the aspirants with varieties of question and answer which will satisfy the need of the hour. The editor would feel amply rewarded, if the book satisfy the requirements of the aspirants.

For further improvement of this book suggestion and comments for the esteemed readers are highly solicited to make it a torch bearer to the readers in the concerned field.

Dr. Samik Kumar Paul

Contents

Chief Editor/Author

Chief Editor

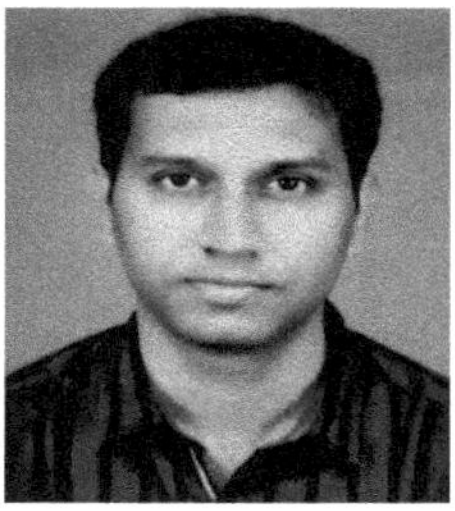

Dr. Samik Kumar Paul started his professional career as Veterinary Officer under Govt. of West Bengal in the year 2010. Presently Dr. Paul is working as Assistant Director, ARD, (Veterinary Research and Investigation),Govt. of West Bengal. The author did his M.V.Sc in Animal Nutrition from West Bengal University of Animal and Fishery Sciences,in 2006, served as Senior Research Fellow under A.I.C.R.P from 2007 to 2009. He has published several research papers in various reputed international and national journals. Dr. Paul is the life member of the association APHV and IVA.

Co-Authors

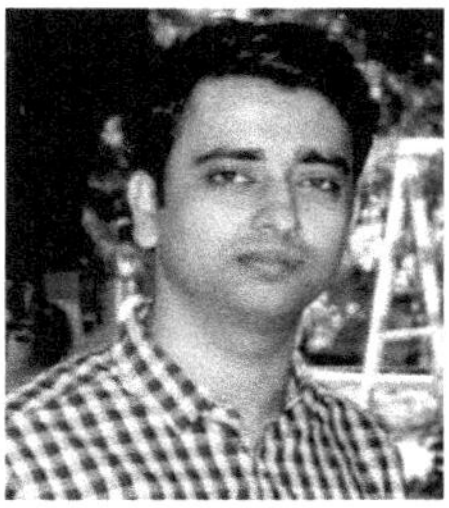

Dr. Sougat Chakrabarty, presently working as Assistant Director, ARD, (Fodder), Govt. of West Bengal. The author started his career as Veterinary Officer in Royal Calcutta Turf Club. Subsequently he joined as Animal Health Officer in FSBS, PBGSBS and Assistant Research Scientist at Amul Research and Development Association. Dr. Chakrabarty was awarded Gold Medal from West Bengal University of Animal and Fishery Sciences for his academic excellence. He is a life member of the Association of Public Health Veterinarian, and Convenor of Indian Veterinary Association (Youth wing), West Bengal.

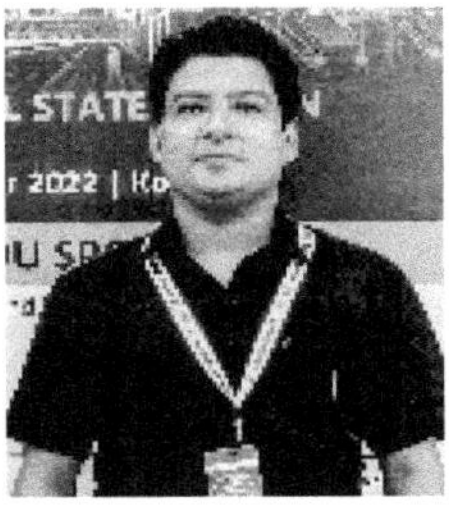

Dr. Probhakar Biswas started his professional career as Veterinary Officer under Govt. of West Bengal in 2009. Subsequently he served as Block Livestock Development Officer. Presently Dr. Biswas is working as Assistant Professor Dept. of Avian Sciences, West Bengal University of Animal and Fishery Sciences (WBUAFS), Kolkata. The author did his PhD in Livestock Production Management form Indian Veterinary Research Institute, Bareilly, U.P in the year 2014. He has published several book chapters and scientific research papers in national and international Journals of repute. He has earned several academic recognitions.

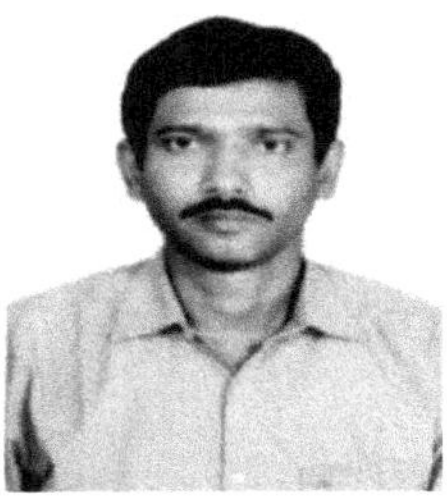

Dr. Arun Kumar Mandal started his professional career as Assistant Professor in Dept. of Anatomy, College of Veterinary Sc. and A.H., O.U.A.T., Bhubaneswar in 2002. Subsequently he joined as Associate Professor in Dept. of Veterinary Anatomy and Histology, F/O-Veterinary and Animal Sciences, West Bengal University of Animal and Fishery Sciences (WBUAFS), Kolkata in 2016. Presently Dr. Mandal has been serving as Professor w.e.f. 2019 in the same Dept. The author has published more than eighty (80) scientific research papers in national and international Journals of repute. He has earned several academic and professional recognitions.

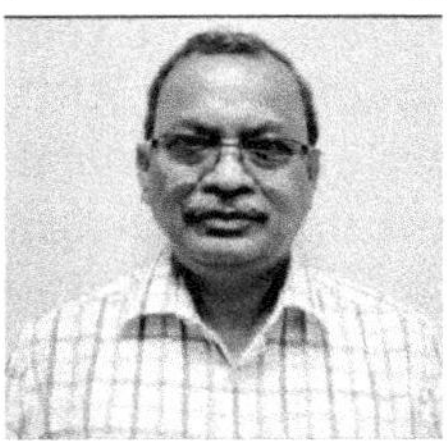

Dr. Tapan Sadhukhan is an eminent veterinary microbiologist, started his carrier as Training Assistant in K.V.K, Nimpith in the year 1986. He retired from service as Joint Director, ARD, West Bengal in the year 2021. He has published several research articles n various reputed International and National journals.

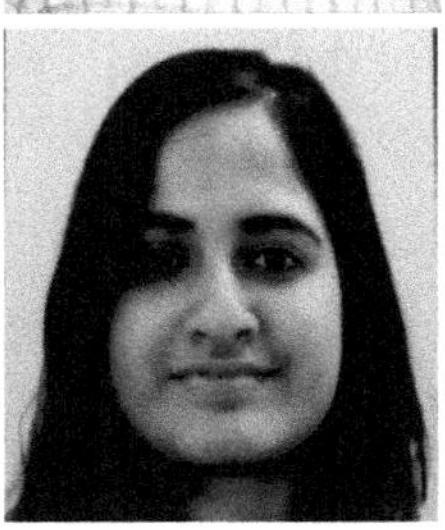

Dr. Ratanti Sarkhel, presently working as Scientist, CSIR- Indian Institute of Chemical Biology. She started her career as Veterinary Officer, under Govt of West Bengal. She awarded Gold Medal from West Bengal University of Animal and Fishery Sciences for her academic excellence. She did her M.V.Sc and PhD form Indian Veterinary Research Institute, Bareilly, U.P. She has published several research papers in SCI indexed journals.

Chapter 1

Veterinary Anatomy

1. **What are the number of skeletal segments in different animals and fowl/bird?**

   Answer:

Animal	*Skull*	*Vertebral Column*	*Ribs, Sternum and Clavicle*	*Fore Limb*	*Hind limb*	*Visceral Bone*	*Total*
Cattle	32	51	26+1+0	24x2	24x2	2 os cordis	208
Horse	32	51	36+1+0	20x2	20x2	-	200
Dog	32	51	26+1+2	44x2	45x2	1 os penis	291
Pig	30	52	(28-30)+1+0	40x2	40x2	1 os rostrale	274
Fowl	40	41	14+1+1+2	13x2 (with coracoids)	21x2	2 os opticus	169

2. **What are the major bones of pectoral limb/fore limb**

   Answer:

   A. Scapula
   B. Humerus
   C. Radius and Ulna
   D. Carpus (carpals)
   E. Metacarpus (Large and Small metacarpals)

F. Phalanges (1st, 2nd and 3rd)

G. Proximal and distal sesamoids

3. What are the major bones of hind limb/pelvic limb?

Answer:

A. Pelvic bones or os coxae:

  a. Ilium

  b. Ischium

  c. Pubis

B. Femur

C. Patella

D. Tibia and Fibula

E. Tarsus (tarsals)

F. Metatarsus (Large and Small metacarpals)

G. Phalanges (1st, 2nd and 3rd)

H. Proximal and distal sesamoids

4. Mention the joints of the fore limb and bones involved.

Answer:

a. Shoulder joint: Between scapula and the humerus

b. Elbow joint: Between humerus and radius and between radius and ulna.

c. Carpal/knee joint: Between carpal bones and radius and ulna, among carpals and distal carpals with metacarpals

d. Inter metacarpal articulation: Between the metacarpal bones.

e. Fetlock joint: Between metacarpals, first phalanx with proximal sesamoids.

f. Pastern joint: Between first and second phalanges.

g. Coffin joint: Between second and third phalanges with distal sesamoid.

5. Mention the joints of the hind limb with the bones involved

Answer:

a. Sacro-iliac joint: Between the articular surfaces of ilium and sacrum.

b. Pelvic symphysis: Between pubis and ischium of two sides (right and left os coxae)

c. Hip joint: Between the acetabulum of os coxae and head of the femur.

d. Stifle joint: Between femur, tibia and patella

e. Tibio fibular joint: Between tibia and fibula

f. Hock joint: Between tibia and tarsal bones, among tarsals and distal tarsals with metatarsals

g. Fetlock joint: Between metatarsal and first phalanx with proximal sesamoids.

h. Pastern joint: Between first and second phalanges.

i. Coffin joint: Between second and third phalanges with distal sesamoid.

6. Where is the mental foramen present?

Answer: Mandible

7. Which are the pneumatic bones in fowl?

Answer: Sternum and humerus

8. Foramen triosseum is formed in —

Answer: Bird

9. The smallest bone is —

Answer: Stapes (middle ear)

10. Ring bone is commonly found in

Answer: Horse (pastern or coffin joint)

11. Largest long bone of the skeleton in animals is

Answer: Femur

12. What is cannon bone?

Answer: Large metacarpal/metatarsal bone in horse

13. Which are the splint bones?

Answer: Small metacarpal/metatarsal bones in horse

14. What is pin bone?

Answer: Tuber ischii (ischial tuberosity) of ischium none is referred as pin bone.

15. What is point of hip?

Answer: External angle of ilium (tuber coxae)

16. In which species is synsacrum formed?

Answer: Avian (birds)

17. Which bones form pelvic cavity/bony pelvis?

Answer: Os-coxae, sacrum and first 2-3 coccygeal vertebra

18. In which species supra-condyloid fossa(femur) is absent?

Answer: Dog

19. Which one is the largest foramen of the body (in animals)?

Answer: Obturator foramen (or coxae)

20. Hip bones are also known as

Answer: Os coxae/pelvic bones/coxal bones/innominate bones

21. Which measurements are usually associated with pelvimetry in animals?

Answer: Conjugate diameter and transverse diameter

22. In which species pelvic symphysis is absent?

Answer: Fowl/bird

23. In which domestic animal 3rd trochanter (femur) is present?

Answer: Horse

24. Which one is the largest sesamoid bone?

Answer: Patella

25. What is the shape of patella in cattle, horse and dog?

Answer: cattle- triangular, horse – almost square shaped (blunt apex), dog – oval

26. Which structure characterizes sexual dimorphism in tarsometatarsus bone of fowl?

Answer: In male birds presence of conical bony spur at distal 3rd part of the bone

27. Pituitary/hypophyseal fossa is also called as

Answer: Sella turcica (sphenoid bone)

28. Cephalic Index is associated with the following parts of the body

Answer: It indicates the shape of the skull

29. What is the bony structure of horn in domestic ruminants?

Answer: Cornual process of frontal bone

30. Which is the largest foramen in skull of domestic animals?

Answer: Foramen magnum

31. Name the bones that form upper jaw of domestic animals.

Answer: Maxilla and premaxilla

32. What is trephining of skull?

Answer: Surgical opening/perforation into the skull sinuses

33. Name the structure through which stomach tube is inserted in horse.

Answer: Ventral nasal meatus (nose)

34. Name the types of skulls in dogs.

Answer: Brachycephalic (short and wide), Dolichocephalic (long and narrow), mesaticephalic (intermediate type)

35. Which bone forms point of the elbow?

Answer: Olecranon process of the ulna

36. What is the point of hock?

Answer: Tuber calcis/calcaneal tuber of fibular tarsal (attachment site of Achilles tendon)

37. Acromion process, spine, glenoid cavity, *etc.* are parts of -

Answer: Scapula (shoulder bone/shoulder blade/pectoral girdle)

38. Hardest structure in an animal body is

Answer: Enamel

39. Furculum is a part of

Answer: clavicle bone of fowl

40. What is os-cordis?

Answer: The supporting tissues of cardiac valves consist of fibrous ring (annuli fibrosi) that surrounds the atrio-ventricular and arterial orifices of the heart and is observed in large ruminants like cattle, water buffaloes.

41. Epidural anesthesia in cows is generally given in between -

Answer: 1st and 2nd coccygeal vertebra

42. Which bone is called Atlas?

Answer: First cervical vertebra

43. Which is the longest vertebra?

Answer: Second cervical vertebra (Axis)

44. What is loin in domestic animals?

Answer: Lumbar area

45. **Which body part is called rump?**

Answer: Sacral area

46. **What is pygostyle?**

Answer: Prismatic mass formed by fused coccygeal vertebrae in fowl/bird

47. **In which type of angular movement, the angle is reduced?**

Answer: Flexion

48. **What are archiform ligaments?**

Answer: Arch shaped ligaments connecting corresponding aspect of proximal ends of radius and ulna is called archiform ligaments

49. **Give an example of hinge joint**

Answer: Humero- radial/femoro-tibial joint

50. **Which joint is called pastern joint?**

Answer: Proximal inter-phalangeal joint

51. **Distal interphalangeal joint is also known as -**

Answer: Coffin joint

52. **Cruciate ligaments(cattle) are present in —**

Answer: Stifle and coffin joint

53. **The horses can't sidekick due to presence of —**

Answer: Accessory ligament (in addition to round ligament) in hip joint (so hip dislocation is less common in this animal)

54. **What is nucleus pulposus?**

Answer: Soft center of intervertebral disc. Slipped disc is due to protrusion of this soft portion.

55. **The ligaments connecting the arches of the adjacent vertebra**

Answer: Ligamentum flava

56. **Which ligament is characteristic of grazing animals?**

Answer: Nuchal ligament/ligamentum nuchae

57. **What are he check ligaments?**

Answer: In case of equine/horse, superior and inferior check ligaments of the limbs are connected with SDF and DDF tendons respectively and help prevent/check flexion of digital joints

58. What is ligamentum nuchae?

Answer: cervical continuation of supraspinous ligament is known as ligamentum nuchae.

59. Which ligament is surgically cut in MPD operation in domestic animals?

Answer: Medial straight patellar ligament

60. Name a pivot/trochoid joint (with rotation movement).

Answer: Atlanto-axial joint

61. What is suspensory ligament in limbs of the domestic animals?

Answer: Modified interosseous muscle, otherwise called superior sesamoidean ligament, closely adhered with the posterior aspect of large metacarpal/metatarsal bone and help support the digital joints, specifically fetlock.

62. Why can a horse stand for a much longer time or even sleep in standing position?

Answer: Due to the supporting system of suspensory apparatus (both limbs) and reciprocal apparatus (hindlimb)

63. What are the muscles of the thorax and abdomen?

Answer:

Thoracic muscles

a. External intercostals
b. Internal intercostals
c. Retractor costarum (partly)
d. Rectus thoracis
e. Transversus thoracis
f. Serratus thoracis (dorsalis and ventralis)
g. Latissimus dorsi
h. Diaphragm
g. Longissimus costarum and levator costarum

Abdominal muscles

a. Obliquus abdominis externus (wall)
b. Obliquus abdominis internus (wall)
c. Rectus abdominis (floor)
d. Transversus abdominis (wall)

64. Give an example of cruciate muscle

Answer: Masseter muscle (face)

65. Name one spiral muscle.

Answer: Brachialis (arm)

66. Name two straight muscles.

Answer: Rectus abdominis and rectus femoris

67. Name the longest and strongest muscle of the animal body.

Answer: Longissimus dorsi

68. Name the usual site of I/M injection in domestic animals.

Answer: Gluteus muscle (hip)

69. How jugular groove/furrow in neck is formed?

Answer: between brachiocephalicus dorsally and sternocephalicus ventrally

70. What is pennate muscle?

Answer: Muscle with feather-like arrangement of muscle fibers (*e.g.* Gastrocnemius)

71. What is diaphragm?

Answer: Dome shaped musculo-tendinous partition between thoracic and abdominal cavity, the chief inspiratory muscle

72. Diaphragm is rudimentary or absent in –

Answer: Bird/fowl

73. Which muscle forms hump in Zebu cattle?

Answer: Rhomboideus (along with fatty tissue)

74. What is hamstring?

Answer: The posterior femoral muscles (biceps femoris, semitendinosus and semimembranosus) are called as hamstring (which extend the hock joint).

75. What is inguinal canal?

Answer: There is potential oblique space/passage between internal and external oblique muscles of the abdomen on either side for passage of testis/ spermatic cord, related blood vessels, nerves, round ligament of uterus *etc.* It is the site of inguinal hernia.

76. Which is the largest flight muscle in a bird?

Answer: Pectoralis/breast muscle

77. What is brisket region in animals?

Answer: Protrusion/prominence formed by pectoral muscles between two forelimbs

78. What is rump muscle?

Answer: Gluteus and ilio-psoas muscles

79. What is capped elbow and capped hock condition?

Answer: Pathological condition (chronic inflammation/bursitis) of olecranon bursa (at olecranon process of ulna/point of elbow) and calcaneal bursa (at tuber calcis/point of hock) respectively

80. The hyoid muscles involved in elevation of tongue is

Answer: Mylohyoideus

81. Falx Cerebri, tentorium cerebelli and diaphragm sellae are infoldings of

Answer: Dura mater(cranial)

82. The balance of the body is controlled by which part of the brain?

Answer: Cerebellum

83. What is rhinencephalon?

Answer: Parts of telencephalon (fore brain) associated with the sense of smell

84. Which of the domestic animals possesses most acute sense of smell (macrosmatic)?

Answer: Dog

85. What are the ventricles of brain?

Answer: Lateral ventricles (right and left), 3rd ventricle and 4th ventricle

86. Name the pathological condition associated with blockage of CSF circulation inside brain.

Answer: Hydrocephalus

87. What is sensory relay center of brain?

Answer: Thalamus

88. Name the brain structure wherefrom material/tissue is collected for Rabies diagnosis.

Answer: Hippocampus

89. Name the site of CSF formation.

Answer: Choroid plexus (ventricles of brain)

90. What is the common site of CSF collection?

Answer: Cisterna magna

91. Name the largest commissure of the brain.

Answer: Corpus callosum

92. Which species have smooth surfaced cerebrum?

Answer: Fowl/bird

93. What is the connection of lateral ventricles with 3rd ventricle of brain?

Answer: Foramen of Monro

94. Name the part of brain having vermis lobe.

Answer: Cerebellum

95. Which part of brain is associated with emotion?

Answer: Amygdala

96. What are the parts of diencephalon (inter brain)?

Answer: Thalamus, epithalamus, hypothalamus, metathalamus, subthalamus and 3rd ventricle

97. What are the parts of mesencephalon (mid brain)?

Answer: 4 colliculi, 2 cerebral peduncles, cerebral aqueduct and inter peduncular fossa

98. Name the part of brain containing vital centers of respiration, circulation, swallowing and vomition

Answer: Medulla oblongata

99. Name the posterior tapering end of spinal cord.

Answer: Conus medullaris (with cauda equina arrangement of spinal nerves)

100. Name the meninges covering in domestic animals.

Answer: Duramater, arachnoid and piamater (from outside inward)

101. Which is the largest cranial nerve?

Answer: Trigeminal nerve (5th)

102. Which is the longest cranial nerve?

Answer: Vagus nerve (10th)

103. Which one is the smallest cranial nerve?

Answer: Trochlear nerve (4th)

104. Cornual nerve is a branch of-

Answer: Trigeminal (ophthalmic branch) nerve

105. The largest nerve in an animal's body is -

Answer: Sciatic nerve

106. Name the nerve associated with facial paralysis.

Answer: Dorsal buccal nerve (branch of facial nerve)

107. What causes dropped elbow in domestic animals?

Answer: Damage to radial nerve

108. In which domestic animal obturator paralysis is common?

Answer: Cattle(cow)

109. Name the nerve innervating external genital organs.

Answer: Pudental nerve

110. Which nervous system is involuntary in nature?

Answer: Autonomic nervous system (ANS)

111. What is tusk of elephant?

Answer: Upper 2nd incisor teeth

112. What is tusk of pig?

Answer: Canine teeth

113. Name the cranial nerves, mention their type and distribution

Answer:

Sl.No.	*Name*	*Type*	*Distribution*
1	Olfactory	Sensory	Nasal mucosa (Smell)
2	Optic	Sensory	Retina of eye(sight)
3	Oculomotor	Motor	Eye muscles (most)
4	Trochlear	Motor	Eye muscle (dorsal oblique)
5	Trigeminal	Mixed	Skin of upper face, jaw, ear, tongue, gums, palate, nasal cavity, teeth and muscles of mastication
6	Abducens	Motor	Lateral rectus and retractor oculi muscles of eye
7	Facial	Mixed	Facial muscles, ear and anterior 2/3 rd of tongue (taste buds)

Sl.No.	Name	Type	Distribution
8.	Auditory/cochleo-vestibular	Sensory	Internal ear (cochlea, vestibule, semicircular canals)(Hearing and equilibrium/balance)
9	Glossopharyngeal	Mixed	Posterior 1/3 rd of tongue (taste buds), muscles of pharynx and parotid gland
10	Vagus	Mixed	Pharynx, larynx, heart, trachea, lungs, oesophagus, stomach and other abdominal viscera
11	Spinal accessory	Motor	Sternomastoideus and trapezius muscles (neck and shoulder)
12	Hypoglossal	Motor	Intrinsic and extrinsic muscles of tongue

114. Name the nerves originating from Brachial plexus and mention the region supplied.

Answer: Brachial Plexus branches/nerves and innervation

Nerve	*Region Supplied*
External thoracic	Shoulder, thoracic, abdominal (skin)
Thoracodorsal	Shoulder
Pectoral	Shoulder
Long thoracic	Shoulder
Subscapular	Shoulder
Suprascapular	Shoulder
Axillary	Shoulder
Musculo cutaneous	Arm
Radial	Arm and forearm and even digit
Ulnar	Forearm and digit
Median	Forearm and digit

115. Which teeth erupt very late and are never replaced?

Answer: Molar teeth

116. What is frenum linguae?

Answer: Mucous fold connecting ventral surface of tongue with oral floor

117. What is the peculiar shape of tongue apex tip in horse?

Answer: Spatula like

118. Name the nerves originating from Lumbosacral plexus and mention the region supplied.

Answer: Lumbosacral plexus branches/nerves and innervation.

Nerve	*Region Supplied*
Cranial gluteal	Rump
Caudal gluteal	Rump
Femoral nerve	Thigh
Obturator nerve	Thigh
Ischiatic/Sciatic	Thigh
Tibial	Leg, digit
Common peroneal	Leg, digit

119. In which species torus linguae and fossa linguae are present?

Answer: Tongue of ruminants

120. What is lyssa?

Answer: In canine tongue, a fibro-muscular cord like structure present ventro-medially at apex, called lyssa

121. Which part of ruminant stomach shows internally Honey comb like structure?

Answer: Reticulum

122. Which chamber of ruminant stomach internally appears like Turkish towel?

Answer: Rumen

123. Name one ruminant without omasum in stomach.

Answer: Camel

124. The largest salivary gland in cattle is —

Answer: Parotid.

125. The zygomatic salivary gland is found in —

Answer: Dog

126. Name the domestic animal having the largest caecum.

Answer: Horse

127. Characteristic spiral colon is seen in –

Answer: Ruminants and pig

128. What is margoplicatus?

Answer: Ridge like mucosal separation between non glandular and glandular part of equine stomach

129. Name the stomach in fowl/bird.

Answer: Glandular- proventriculus, muscular – gizzard

130. Name the parts of cloaca in bird/fowl.

Answer: Coprodeum, urodeum and proctodeum (with dorsal connection of bursa of Fabricius)

131. What is Vermiform appendix?

Answer: Terminal, narrow part of caecum

132. Remnant of yolk sac present in jejunum of fowl/bird is called as

Answer: Meckel's diverticulum

133. What is Stenson's duct?

Answer: Duct or parotid gland.

134. What is Wharton's duct?

Answer: Mandibular gland duct

135. What is the site of ruminal motility counting?

Answer: Left para lumbar fossa (by palpation)

136. Name the largest solid gland of the animal body.

Answer: Liver

137. What is the largest attachment/ligament of liver?

Answer: Falciform ligament (on parietal surface of liver with diaphragm)

138. In which species of domestic animal gall bladder is absent?

Answer: Horse/equine

139. How liver of dog and pig is oriented?

Answer: Transversely across the median plane

140. In TRP case, which operation is carried out?

Answer: Rumenotomy

141. The Vomeronasal organ is also known as

Answer: Organ of Jacobson

142. False nostril (nasal diverticulum) is present in —

Answer: Horse

143. Signet ring shaped cartilage in front of first tracheal ring

Answer: Cricoid cartilage

144. Which one is the largest cartilage of larynx?

Answer: Thyroid cartilage

145. What is glottis?

Answer: The narrow vertical space between two vocal cords

146. The number of lobes in the left and right lungs of cattle is

Answer: Left - 3, Right- 4(additional accessory lobe)

147. Name the sound producing organ in birds/fowl.

Answer: Syrinx (at tracheal bifurcation)

148. Name the largest air sac of fowl/bird.

Answer: Abdominal air sac (out of usually 8 air sacs)

149. Name the additional bronchus for apical lobe of right lung (cattle and pig).

Answer: Apical/tracheal bronchus

150. What is mediastinum?

Answer: The inter-pleural space between two pleural sacs/lungs

151. What is the usual location of kidneys in domestic animals and birds?

Answer: Lumbar area and lumbar and pelvic area, respectively

152. Which kidney in domestic animals is variable in position?

Answer: Left kidney (due to varying degree of fullness of stomach)

153. The shape of the kidneys in domestic animals and birds are –

Answer: Small ruminants, dog, pig- bean shaped, cattle – bean (right), pyramidal/3 sided (left), horse – heart shaped (right), bean shaped (left), birds – elongated

154. Lobated kidneys are characteristic of following domestic animal –

Answer: Large ruminant (cattle/buffalo)

155. Non lobated kidneys are characteristic of following domestic animal –

Answer: Small ruminants, dog, pig, horse

156. What is the site of urinary bladder puncture in dog, small ruminants and pig?

Answer: Prepubic area (along midline)

157. Why catheterization of urinary bladder is difficult in bull and boar?

Answer: Due to presence of sigmoid flexure of penis and dorsal diverticulum of urethra (for ducts of bulbourethral gland)

158. What is the position of testes and scrotum in different domestic animals?

Answer: Cattle, horse – inguinal, dog, pig – close to anus

159. Which domestic animals are characterized by presence of Os-penis?

Answer: Dog and cat

160. Name the domestic animal with tail of epididymis facing upward.

Answer: Pig/boar

161. Urethral process is best developed in –

Answer: Small ruminants

162. Corona glandis, urethral sinus, fossa glandis are observed in –

Answer: Penis of horse

163. Cork screw like penis and preputial diverticulum characteristic of –

Answer: Pig/boar

164. What is the surgical removal of testis called?

Answer: castration

165. In which species Bulbourethral glands and seminal vesicles are absent?

Answer: Dog (only Prostate gland is present)

166. Mature ovary appears like a bunch of grapes in –

Answer: Hen/bird

167. Ovulation fossa is located on the ovary of

Answer: Mare

168. Body of uterus is longest in –

Answer: Mare

169. Jejunum coil like uterine horn is seen in –

Answer: Sow

170. Almost Y or V shaped uterus is observed in –

Answer: Bitch

171. Uterine caruncles are characteristic of –

Answer: Cow/bovine

172. Sub urethral diverticulum is clinically important in –

Answer: Cow and sow

173. What is the shape of area of auscultation and percussion of lungs?

Answer: Roughly triangular (posterior angle of scapula to last inter costal space dorsally with third point close to point of elbow ventrally)

174. Which chamber forms the apex of heart?

Answer: Left ventricle

175. What is SA node/pace maker of heart?

Answer: The site of right atrium (close to cranial vena cava) that generates and conducts the nerve impulse for autonomic/intrinsic, rhythmic contraction of heart muscle

176. What is the usual area of auscultation of heart in domestic animals?

Answer: 4th and 5th inter costal space on left side

177. What is mitral valve of heart?

Answer: Bicuspid valves guarding the left atrio-ventricular opening (resembling Bishop's mitre/cap)

178. What is the blood supply to heart itself?

Answer: By coronary arteries (right and left)

179. Name the location of semilunar valves in heart.

Answer: At the origin of aorta (from left ventricle) and pulmonary trunk (from right ventricle)

180. Name the attachment of apex of heart in domestic animals.

Answer: Cattle and horse- pericardiaco- sternal ligaments, dog – pericardiaco-phrenic ligaments (due to much inclined apex close to diaphragm)

181. The artery associated with blood supply to diaphragm is

Answer: Phrenic artery

182. Which artery supplies stomach and associated structures?

Answer: Coeliac artery

183. Name the main arteries supplying forelimbs and hindlimbs of domestic animals.

Answer: Forelimb – Axillary/Brachial artery, Hindlimb – External iliac artery

184. Name the artery supplying structures of pelvic cavity in domestic animals.

Answer: Internal iliac artery

185. Name the artery supplying most of the intestine in domestic animals.

Answer: Anterior/cranial mesenteric artery

186. What is the arterial supply of brain in domestic animals?

Answer: Branches from Circle of Willis

187. The preferred artery for recording pulse in large ruminants?

Answer: Middle coccygeal artery (ventral part of the base of the tail).

188. Which is the preferred artery for recording the pulse in small ruminants and dog?

Answer: Femoral/saphenous artery (medial aspect of thigh)

189. What are the bypass channels in foetal circulation?

Answer: Ductus venosus, foramen ovale and ductus arteriosus

190. How milk veins are useful in high yielding cows?

Answer: Milk veins (subcutaneous abdominal veins) become very prominent and tortuous

191. Which artery and nerve are taken care of during dehorning operation?

Answer: Ligation of cornual artery and blocking of cornual nerve

192. For I/V infusion or injection which vein is used in different animals?

Answer:

- ☆ Cattle and Horse: Jugular Vein (external jugular vein)
- ☆ Pig: Ear vein,
- ☆ Dog: Radial/cephalic vein (fore limb) and Recurrent tarsal vein (hind limb)

193. What is the lymph reservoir in animal body?

Answer: Cisterna chyli

194. Name the largest lymphatic channel of the body.

Answer: Thoracic duct

195. Name some superficial (palpable) lymph nodes of domestic animals.

Answer: Parotid LN, mandibular LN, prescapular LN, prefemoral LN *etc.*

196. Which is the largest lymph node of the body?

Answer: Posterior mediastinal.

197. In which animals haemal nodes are present?

Answer: Ruminants

198. The largest lymphoid organ (in animals) is —

Answer: Spleen

199. There is absence of true lymph nodes in —

Answer: Chicken and Turkey.

200. The largest organ of the body is

Answer: Skin

201. What is frog?

Answer: Wedge shaped structure between bars on the solar part of the hoof in horse

202. What are ergots?

Answer: Rudimentary/vestigial digits on posterior surface of fetlock joints in horse

203. What is coronary band?

Answer: A narrow band of soft tissue around the coronary border of hoof at the junction of hoof and skin

204. The third eyelid (nictating membrane) is well developed in —

Answer: Horse, camel, cat and bird

205. Cataract is associated with—

Answer: Lens of eye

206. Colour of eye is determined by –

Answer: Iris

207. What is tapetum lucidum?

Answer: Reflecting medium of eye (choroid) and best developed in nocturnal animals like cat

208. White of the eye is formed by –

Answer: Sclera

209. Yellow spot (most acute vision) and blind spot (least vision) are present in –

Answer: Retina

210. During extirpation/removal of eye ball following structures are cut –

Answer: 7 ocular muscles, optic nerve, blood vessels and periorbita

211. Name the cartilages of external ear.

Answer: Annular, conchal and scutiform cartilages

212. Haematoma condition usually affects –

Answer: External ear flap

213. Ear ossicles (malleus, incus and stapes) are present in –

Answer: Middle ear (stapes, the smallest bone)

214. Guttural pouches (pouch like dilatation of pharyngeal end of auditory tube) are observed in

Answer: Horse

215. Why pinna is movable in domestic animals?

Answer: Due to the presence of extrinsic auricular muscles

216. Name the muscles of middle ear.

Answer: Tensor tympani and stapedius

217. Where internal ear is present?

Answer: Within petrous temporal bone (hardest bone of the body)

218. Saccule, utricle and semi-circular canals are part of –

Answer: Vestibule (internal ear)

219. Organ of sense of hearing is –

Answer: Spiral organ/organ of Corti (cochlea of internal ear)

220. What is aesthesiology?

Answer: Study of sense organs/system

221. Suprarenal gland is otherwise known as –

Answer: Adrenal gland

222. Endocrine gland associated with larynx and trachea of domestic animals is –

Answer: Thyroid gland

223. Posterior pituitary stores and releases –

Answer: Oxytocin and vasopressin/ADH

224. How gut/GI hormones act?

Answer: They act locally in a particular gut segment and influence gut motility

225. What are the basic tissues of the body?

Answer: Epithelium, connective tissue, muscular tissue and nervous tissue

226. What is mesothelium?

Answer: Simple squamous epithelium lining serous membrane

227. What is endothelium?

Answer: Simple squamous epithelium lining the lumen of blood vessels

228. What is urothelium?

Answer: Transitionale epithelium of urinary tracts, *etc.*

229. Glandular epithelium is –

Answer: Modified simple cuboidal epithelium

230. What is the epithelium of esophagus, rumen, reticulum and omasum of cattle?

Answer: Stratified squamous epithelium (keratinized)

231. Epithelium of glandular stomach, gall bladder, small intestine and large intestine (most part) is-

Answer: Simple columnar epithelium

232. Name the cell processes.

Answer: Microvilli, cilia, flagella and stereocilia

233. Brush border epithelium is seen in –

Answer: small intestine, PCT of nephron *etc.*

234. Pseudostratified columnar epithelium is commonly seen in –

Answer: Respiratory tract (trachea, bronchus *etc.*) and epididymis.

235. What is unicellular mucus secreting gland?

Answer: Goblet cell

236. Name the common glands of skin.

Answer: Sweat gland, sebaceous gland

237. Name one mixed type of gland.

Answer: Pancreas (exocrine acini and endocrine islets of Langerhans)

238. Name some compound glands.

Answer: Salivary glands, mammary glands, male accessory sex glands *etc.*

239. Name one cytogenous glands.

Answer: Testis/ovary

240. Name the connective tissue fibers.

Answer: Collagen, elastic and reticular fibers

241. Name some connective tissue cells.

Answer: Fibroblast/fibrocyte, plasma cell, macrophage, reticular cells, mast cell, adipocytes, leukocytes *etc.*

242. Name the cells of bone and cartilages.

Answer: Bone – osteoblast, osteocyte (mature), osteoclast(phagocyte), cartilage – chondroblast, chondrocyte(mature)

243. What are Haversian canals?

Answer: There are numerous very narrow canals that pass through the compact substance along the length of the bone are known as Haversian canals.

244. What are Volkmann's canals?

Answer: The Haversian canals communicate with the marrow cavity and with surface of the bones by some transverse canals which are not surrounded by bony lamella.

245. Characteristic dark and light bands are seen in –

Answer: Skeletal and cardiac muscles (striated)

246. Involuntary muscles are –

Answer: Smooth muscle and cardiac muscle

247. What is sarcomere?

Answer: Contractile unit of striated muscle between 2 adjacent Z lines

248. Name the major muscle filaments.

Answer: Actin and myosin

249. What are the principal cells of nervous system.

Answer: Neurons and glial cells

250. Name the largest and smallest glial cells.

Answer: largest – astrocyte, smallest- microglia (phagocytic)

251. Glial cells lining the brain ventricles and central canal of spinal cord is –

Answer: Ependyma

252. How many cell layers constitute the cerebral cortex of animals?

Answer: Six

253. Number of cell layers in cerebellar cortex is –

Answer: Three

254. Purkinje cells are present in

Answer: Cerebellum (cortex)

255. Pyramidal cells are present in –

Answer: Cerebral cortex

256. Which part of neuron forms the nerve fiber?

Answer: Axon

257. Name the routine histological staining method.

Answer: Haematoxylin and eosin (H and E)

258. Name the tissue sectioning machine/instrument.

Answer: Microtome

259. What is ultrastructural study?

Answer: Detailed study of cellular structure by electron microscope (TEM)

260. Microscope used for routine histological study is

Answer: Compound light microscope

261. Name the lingual papillae with taste buds.

Answer: fungiform, vallet and foliate papillae (gustatory)

262. Name mechanical papillae.

Answer: Filiform, lenticular and conical papillae

263. What is the arrangement of intrinsic tongue muscles?

Answer: Longitudinal, transverse and vertical

264. Name the main cell population in fundic (gastric) glands.

Answer: Chief cells, parietal cells and mucous neck cells

265. What are crypts of Lieberkuhn?

Answer: These are simple tubular intestinal glands between the villi base

266. What is goblet cell population in intestinal epithelium?

Answer: Number of goblet cells increases caudally from small towards large intestine

267. What are the histological layers of any tubular structure?

Answer: Inner mucosa surrounded by submucosa, tunica muscularis/ muscular and serosa/adventitia

268. What are intestinal villi?

Answer: Finger like microscopic structural modifications of small intestinal mucosa (animals)

269. Brunner's glands in animals are usually present in

Answer: Duodenum (submucosa)

270. Peyer's patches are present in the wall of -

Answer: Ileum

271. Anal glands and sacs are characteristic of –

Answer: Dog

272. Macrophages of liver are –

Answer: Kupffer cells

273. Histological unit of liver is –

Answer: Liver/hepatic lobule

274. Typical hexagonal liver lobules are seen in –

Answer: Pig

275. Dentine is produced by —

Answer: Odontoblast cells

276. Type of tracheal/bronchial cartilage is –

Answer: Hyaline

277. Types of cells in lung alveoli are –

Answer: Type I and II pneumocytes, alveolar macrophages (dust cells)

278. What is the structural and functional unit of kidney?

Answer: Nephron

279. Which cells help in glomerular filtration?

Answer: glomerular endothelium and podocytes

280. The thinnest tubular part of nephron is –

Answer: Loop of Henle

281. Testosterone secreting cells of seminiferous epithelium are –

Answer: Interstitial cells/Leydig cells

282. Supporting cells for spermatogenic cells in seminiferous epithelium are –

Answer: Sertoli/sustentacular cells (forming blood-testis barrier)

283. The smallest and largest variety of ovarian follicles in animals are –

Answer: Smallest – primordial follicle, largest – mature/Graafian follicle

284. What is corpus luteum?

Answer: Post ovulation, the follicular cells of the ruptured follicle are reorganized with formation of lutein cells, secreting progesterone required for pregnancy maintenance.

285. What is the external lining of ovary?

Answer: Germinal epithelium

286. During which stages of estrus cycle (in animals) are the uterine/endometrial glands are very well developed?

Answer: During estrus and mete-strus (maximum)

287. What type of gland is mammary gland?

Answer: Compound tubulo-alveolar gland/modified sweat gland

288. Thyroid follicles are lined by –

Answer: cuboidal follicular cells

289. What are C cells?

Answer: Parafollicular cells of the thyroid gland secret calcitonin/thyrocalcitonin

290. What is teratology?

Answer: Study of developmental defects/anomalies

291. Who is referred to as the "Father of modern embryology"?

Answer: Von Baer

292. Spermatogenesis and oogenesis involve –

Answer: Both mitosis and meiosis cell divisions

293. What is the product of fertilization?

Answer: Zygote (2n) formation

294. What is cleavage?

Answer: Rapid successive mitosis of zygote without increasing the size of blastomeres

295. What is morula?

Answer: Mulberry fruit like appearance of embryo during early cleavage

296. What is blastula?

Answer: Embryo formed during late cleavage consisting of fluid filled cavity/ blastocoel surrounded by trophoblast layer and inner cell mass

297. What is gastrula?

Answer: Trilaminar embryo consisting of 3 primary germ layers (endoderm, mesoderm and ectoderm)

298. What are the foetal/extraembryonic membranes?

Answer: Yolk sac, amnion, allantois and chorion (outermost)

299. What are the types of placentae in different animals/species?

Answer: Cow- cotyledonary, syndesmochorial, Mare and sow -diffuse, epitheliochorial, Bitch/queen -zonary, endotheliochorial, Human- discoidal, haemochorial, Rabbit – discoidal, haemoendothelial

300. What are the successive stages of kidney development?

Answer: Pronephros, mesonephros and metanephros (mammals and bird)

Chapter 2

Veterinary Gynaecology and Obstetrics

1. **What is the age of puberty for cattle and buffalo?**

   Answer: Indigenous cattle: 24 months

   Exotic/crossbred: 12-15 months

   Buffalo: 24-30 months

2. **Mention estrous cycle in different animal?**

   Answer:

Animal	*Length of Estrous Cycle in Days*	*Length of Estrus in Hours/Days*	*Time of Ovulation*
Cow	21-22 days	18-19 hrs	12-16 hours after end of estrous
Goat	21 days or short	30-40 hrs	30-36 hrs from estrus
Ewe	16-17 days	24-30 hrs	24-30 hrs from beginning of estrus
Sow	19-20 days	48-72 hrs	35 – 45 hrs of estrus
Mare	19-25 days	4-8 days	1-2 days before the end of estrus

3. **In cattle and buffalo what is the time of ovulation?**

   Answer: 12-16 hours after the end of estrous.

4. **What is the optimum time of insemination?**

   Answer: Mid heat (standing heat and 6 hours after first insemination)

5. **What is the average conception rate in Artificial Insemination in India?**

   Answer: 35 per cent in India

6. **What is service requirement per conception?**

   Answer: 1.5-1.75

7. **What is the gestation period in cattle and buffalo?**

   Answer: Cattle: 280-290 days

   Buffalo: 305-318 days

8. **What should be the optimum dry period in cattle and buffalo?**

   Answer: 60 days.

9. **What is the gap between calving to first heat in Cattle and Buffalo?**

   Answer: 40 days.

10. **What is the gap between Calving to conception?**

    Answer: 85 days

11. **What is the length of lactation in cattle and buffalo?**

    Answer: 300 to 305 days.

12. **What is the first service pregnancy rate?**

    Answer: 65 per cent

13. **What is approximate birth weight for cattle and buffalo?**

    Answer: Indigenous: 25 kg

    Crossbred: 25-35 kg

    Buffalo: 30-40 kg

14. **Cutaneous lesions resembling ringworms are commonly found in which type of abortion?**

    Answer: Mycotic abortion

15. **Keratinization of the vaginal epithelium, degeneration of the placenta and abortion or dystocia are associated with a deficiency of which vitamin?**

    Answer: Vitamin A

16. Which vitamin is essential for spermatogenesis?

Answer: Vitamin A

17. Uterine torsion is most common in

Answer: Buffalo

18. Uterine torsion is most commonly observed in which trimester?

Answer: Last or 3rd trimester

19. High yielders most frequently suffer from infertility because of

Answer: High level of prolactin, shadowing effect of prolactin on GnRH, limited action of GnRH

20. Peculiar twitching of tail is the indication of

Answer: Uterine torsion

21. Post coital pyometra is seen in

Answer: Trichomoniasis

22. Leathery placenta is the indication of

Answer: Fungal infection

23. Virgin heifer test is associated with diagnosis of

Answer: Campylobacteriosis

24. Long oestrous cycle is seen in case of

Answer: Campylobacteriosis

25. What is the most conducive time to perform artificial insemination in cattle?

Answer: Usually 10-14 hrs after estrous

26. Why should cattle in heat be kept calm before the procedure is performed?

Answer: As long walking or excitement secrets adrenalin hormone which reduce the ciliary movement resulting reduce fertilization process.

27. What is venereal disease? Give some examples in cattle?

Answer: Sexually transmitted disease *e.g.* Brucellosis, Vibriosis, Trichomoniasis

28. What is Anestrus?

Answer: Anestrus can be defined as the lack or absence of the expression of estrus.

29. What are the common methods of semen collection?

Answer: Common methods are-

1. Use of artificial vagina
2. By Electro-stimulation method.
3. By massaging the ampulae of the duct us differences through rectal wall.
4. But the ideal method of semen collection is use of artificial vagina which is safe for sire and the collector also.

30. What are the main causes of anestrus

- ☆ Before puberty – (prepubertal anestrus)
- ☆ After calving – (postpartum anestrus) – Biological protection for dam and offspring
- ☆ Physiological: Hormonal disturbance
- ☆ Nutritional
- ☆ Seasonal (ewe, mare)
- ☆ Pregnancy
- ☆ Anestrous due to different infectious diseases

31. Females of domestic animals reach the puberty at the age of:

- ☆ Mare: 1–2 years
- ☆ Cow: 12-18 months
- ☆ Ewe: 6–15 months
- ☆ Doe or nanny goat: 4–8 months
- ☆ Sow: 6–8 months
- ☆ Bitch: 6–20 months
- ☆ Queen cat: 7–12 months

32. What are the predisposing factors of vaginal prolapse in ruminants?

Answer: The following are said to be predisposing factors:

☆ Hormonal excesses and imbalances ☆ hypocalcaemia ☆ large fetal load (twins or triplets) ☆ fat condition ☆ thin condition ☆ inadequate exercise ☆ short tail docking ☆ bulky food (root crops) ☆ excess dietary fibre ☆ dietary estrogens and their precursors ☆ sloping terrain ☆ vaginal irritation ☆ previous dystocia ☆ inherited predisposition.

33. What are the causes of dystocia in cattle?

- ☆ Fetomaternal disproportion
- ☆ Faulty fetal disposition
- ☆ Incomplete cervical and vaginal dilatation
- ☆ Uterine inertia

- ☆ Uterine torsion
- ☆ Cervical prolapse
- ☆ Pelvic fracture
- ☆ Uterine rupture
- ☆ Cervical neoplasia
- ☆ Fetal abnormalities

34. Name some micronutrients those are required to improve fertility in animals

Answer: Vit-E, Se, Cu, Zn, Mn, Fe, Co and Vit-A

35. What is the gestation period for following animals?

Answer:

- ☆ Cow— 280 days
- ☆ Goat—— 150 days
- ☆ Sow—— 115 days
- ☆ Buffalo—— 310 days
- ☆ Mare— 336 days

36. What are the four steps to be taken to correct the dystocia position?

Answer:

a) Repulsion
b) Rotation
c) Version
d) Adjustment or correction by extension of extremities

37. What are the sources and principal functions of different sex hormones.

Answer:

Hormone	*Source*	*Functions*
Estrogen	Ovary	1. Promotes sexual behavior 2. Development of secondary sex characteristics 3. Anabolism
Progesterone	Luteal cell of Corpus Luteum, placenta and adrenal gland	1. Prepares endometrium for implantation 2. Maintenance of pregnancy
Testosterone	Interstitial cells (Leydig cells) of testis and adrenal cortex	1. Develops and maintains accessory sex glands 2. Stimulates secondary sextual characters and sexual behaviour 3. Controls spermatogenesis process

Hormone	*Source*	*Functions*
Relaxin	Corpus luteum, placenta, uterus	1. Dilatation of cervix and vagina before parturition
Prostaglandin F2	Uterus	1. Causes uterine contraction for smooth transport of spermatozoa 2. Causes luteoysis to regress Corpus luteum 3. Termination of pregnancy

38. What is the procedure or different steps of artificial insemination in cows?

Answer:

a. ***History taking:***

1. When the cattle show estrous signs like bellowing, excited and nervous behavior, mounting to another animal *etc.* Perfect time for AI is in between 12-18hrs from first sign of estrus. So, need to know the history of estrous onset. Considering the fertile life of spermatozoa and ovum the general practice of insemination is to breed the cow in the evening when estrus was first detected in the morning or previous late night. Likewise, cows are bred in the morning when estrus is first detected during the late afternoon in early hrs of night on the previous day.

b. ***Inspection of animal:***

1. Breed of the cow for selecting suitable semen straw. (eg. For upgraded Sahiwal/Gir always Sahiwal/Gir straw should be selected as per breeding policy.)
2. Whether health of the animal is good for AI
3. Animal is still in heat and suitable for AI.
4. In case of disease condition like FMD, Lumpy skin disease *etc.* AI should not be done.
5. In case of any distress condition like walking a long distance during summer *etc.* animal should be kept in crate for ample rest and bathing with cold water should be done before AI.

c. ***AI straw preparation:***

1. After opening the lid of BA-3 can straw filled canister should be drawn up to the neck of the can only.
2. Straw is drawn with vulsellum forcep carefully so that the tip is not broken.
3. Before thawing the straw should be shaken well to remove the traces of LN_2 from the surface of straw. Extra LN_2 from surface of the Straw

is wiped out by cotton. The straw should be completely submerged in horizontal position in warm water during thawing process. Standard method of thawing of frozen semen is to use warm water having temperature 35-37°C. Exposure time of straw to warm water varies from 30 seconds for French mini straw and 45 seconds for French medium straw. Presently used French mini straw (Capacity 0.25ml)

4. After thawing the straw is shaken gently so as to bring air space towards lab seal and is inserted the straw in the AI gun through factory plug, keeping lab seal outer side of the gun.
5. Now the portion of straw containing air space at lab seal is cut at right angle (90°) either by a sharp blade or straw cutter. Next the AI sheath is applied on AI gun.
6. Plunger of gun is pushed forward in such a manner that tip of straw reaches up to anterior part (tip) of sheath and the AI gun is ready for use.
7. The best site of semen deposition is mid/anterior third of cervix and for obtaining better conception rate semen is deposited in form of streak from anterior third to mid cervix.

39. Which frozen semen straw is now generally used for insemination. Mention its capacity, sperm cell concentration and minimum sperm cell post thaw motility.

Answer: French Mini Straw,

Capacity: 0.25ml,

Sperm cell concentration in a straw: 20 million

Minimum sperm cell post thaw Motility: 50 per cent

40. What should be the minimum motility of sperm cells during production of Frozen Semen Straws?

Answer: Minimum motility during production of FSS should be more than 70 per cent.

Chapter 3

Livestock Production Technology

1. **What are the fat percentage of double toned, toned and standardized milk?**

   Answer: 1.5, 3.0, 4.5, respectively

2. **Energy (Kcal) from consumption of 100 gm Cow milk is**

   Answer: 75 Kcal

3. **Fat content in Ghee**

   Answer: 99-99.5 per cent

4. **Calcium phosphorus ratio in milk**

   Answer: Ca:P= 1.24:1

5. **Which exotic breed cow contains highest fat content?**

   Answer: Jersey

6. **Freezing point in case of Mastitis milk**

   Answer: Normal (No change)

7. **Specific gravity of milk fat is**

   Answer: 0.93

8. What is the composition of cow milk and buffalo milk?

Answer:

Constituents	*Concentration (per cent)*	
	Cow Milk	*Buffalo Milk*
Fat	3.6-4.9	6.6-8.8
Protein	3.3-3.5	3.9-4.2
Lactose	4.1-4.5	4.5-5.2
Calcium	0.12	0.18
Phosphorus	0.1	0.1
Magnesium	0.01	0.02
Sodium	0.05	0.04
Potassium	0.15	0.11
Chloride	0.1	0.07

9. Enlist the composition of a whole egg contains

Answer: Moisture 74 per cent, Protein 13 per cent, Fat 11 per cent, Carbohydrate 0.7 per cent, and Ash 1.1 per cent

10. Sweet curdling of milk is due to

Answer: Rennet like enzymes by *Bacillus subtilis*

11. Milk is categorized as A1 or A2 milks based on

Answer: Beta casein

12. Green rot in Eggs on storage is caused by

Answer: *Pseudomonas fluroscence*

13. For good quality egg Haugh unit is

Answer: 72 and above

14. Shelf life of eggs stored at 4°C and 60-70 per cent relative humidity

Answer: 3-4 weeks

15. Pasteurization temperature of egg

Answer: 62-63°C for 3-4 min

16. Which Vitamin is found highest in poultry meat?

Answer: Niacin

17. Which Vitamin is absent in meat

Answer: Vitamin C

18. Ultimate pH of meat is

Answer: 5.5-5.7

19. Brown discoloration of meat is a result of formation of which pigment?

Answer: Metmyoglobin

20. Red spot in Meat is caused by

Answer: Serratia marcescens

21. Musty or earthy flavour in meat is mainly caused by

Answer: Actinomycetes

22. Souring of meat is mainly caused by

Answer: Clostridium sp.

23. Fishy odour in meat is due to

Answer: E. coli

24. Highest egg producing country is

Answer: China

25. Which state produce highest meat in India?

Answer: Uttar Pradesh

26. Average energy value of 100gm buffalo milk is

Answer: 100 Kcal

27. The protein only found in Milk

Answer: Casein

28. The chemical commonly used for meat preservation is

Answer: Citric acid, Benzoic acid and Propionic acid

29. The flavoring agent used in butter is

Answer: Diacetyl

30. Milk is poor source of

Answer: Vitamin C

31. The pH of fresh cow milk is

Answer: 6.4-6.6

32. Meat is a good source of

Answer: Vitamin B

33. The biological value of egg is

Answer: 95 per cent

34. The mineral that helps in precipitation of casein during curdling of milk is

Answer: Calcium

35. Lean meat is almost devoid of

Answer: Vitamin C

36. Pork is rich in

Answer: Thiamine

37. The principal saturated fatty acid present in meat is

Answer: Palmitic acid

38. Commercially sterile meat products are produced by processing meat at

Answer: 100°C

39. Pasteurized meat products are produced by processing meat at

Answer: 58-75°C

40. Average specific gravity of cow milk is

Answer: 1.028-1.030

41. The pH of the buffalo milk is

Answer: 6.7-6.8

42. In which domestic animal fat content is more in milk?

Answer: Ewe

43. Water content is more in the milk of

Answer: Ass

44. Average total solid present in cow milk

Answer: 13 per cent

45. What are the average milk fat percentage of Cow, Buffalo, Sheep, Goat, Camel?

Answer: 4-5 per cent, 7-8 per cent, 7-8 per cent, 3.5-4.5 per cent,2-3 per cent, respectively

46. What are the flush and lean seasons of milk production in West Bengal and India?

Answer: In West Bengal milk flush occurs during the summer (mid of March to mid of August) and remaining months are lean.

In the other states of India milk flush season is winter (November to March) and remaining months are lean.

47. Presence of somatic cells in milk indicates for what?

Answer: Mastitis

48. Marbling appearance in the meat is found due to

Answer: Intramuscular fat

49. Low heat stability of buffalo milk is due to

Answer: Calcium

50. Which enzyme is associated with rancidity of milk?

Answer: Lipase

51. Fresh meat tenderness is assessed by

Answer: Myofibrillar fragmentation Index

52. Main function of salt in a cure mixture is as

Answer: Reducing water activity

53. Name a colour fixing agent used in meat

Answer: Sodium nitrite

54. Rennet used for preparation of cheese contains two principal enzymes namely

Answer: Rennin and Pepsin

55. Neats foot Oil is prepared from

Answer: Cattle hoof

56. Lactose content of cow milk

Answer: 4.1–4.5 per cent

57. Pasteurization efficiency of milk is tested by

Answer: Phosphatase test

58. Operation flood phase 1 is lunched in

Answer: 1970

59. Bacteriological status of milk is judged by

Answer: Dye Reduction Test (MBRT – Methylene Blue Reduction Test)

60. Batch pasteurization is carried out at

Answer: 63°C for 30 minutes (LTHT) or 72°C for 15 sec (HTLT)

61. What is temperature of Ultra heat pasteurization?

Answer: More than 135°C temperature for 2 to 4 sec

62. According to Indian regulations, the permitted maximum number of adult cattle to be transported by road in a vehicle is

Answer: Six

63. What is sliming of intestine

Answer: Removal of mucosa during casing preparation from small intestine.

64. What is Measly beef

Answer: Beef infested with *Cysticercus bovis* is called measly beef.

65. Hormone responsible for letting down of milk

Answer: Oxytocin

66. The predominant protein in egg yolk is

Answer: Ovovitellin

67. Proteins in milk are present as

Answer: Colloidal Suspension

68. What is the pH of freshly drawn milk?

Answer: Slightly Acidic (pH 6.5-6.7)

69. Test for finding the mixing of cow and buffalo milk is

Answer: Hansa test

70. Name an enzyme coagulated dairy product

Answer: Cheese

71. The major component of milk fat

Answer: Triglycerides

72. Young poultry birds reared for eating is called

Answer: Poussins (23-28 days old of age weighing around 0.5 kg)

73. Deer meat is also known as

Answer: Venison

74. Male cattle castrated later in life is called as

Answer: Stag

75. Meat of milk fed calves up to three months of age

Answer: Veal

76. Which Government agency implements AGMARK (Agriculture Marketing)?

Answer: DMI (Directorate of Marketing and Inspection)

77. The autonomous body in India, for certifying quality standards in accordance with international norms

Answer: BIS (Bureau of Indian Standards)

78. Lanolin is obtained from

Answer: Wool of sheep

79. The hormone responsible for holding up of milk

Answer: Adrenalin

80. Name a fermented indigenous dairy product

Answer: Kalan

81. Cow milk is yellowish white in colour while buffalo milk is creamy white, why?

Answer: Cow milk has more β-carotene pigments. In buffalo milk β-carotene pigment gets converted to colourless vitamin A, which makes it less yellowish.

82. In mixed farming system how many per cent of the income must be contributed by the livestock component?

Answer: 10 per cent

83. Milk borne Rickettsial disease

Answer: Q fever

84. Name a pathogen that can multiply under refrigeration temperature

Answer: Listeria

85. Abattoir fever is caused by

Answer: *Coxiella burnetti*

86. Haverhill fever is caused by

Answer: *Streptobacillus moniliformis*

87. Protozoan disease transmitted to man through milk

Answer: Toxoplasmosis

88. Cholinergic drugs can be used to treat ruminal atony true or false?

Answer: Yes, Carbachol is a cholinergic drug primarily used to treat ruminal atony.

89. Antagonist of vitamin K

Answer: Dicumarol

90. Name a phytotoxin

Answer: Ricin present in castor plants

91. An anticoccidial drug that acts by inhibiting Thiamin uptake

Answer: Amprolium

92. Name a non-narcotic anaesthetic

Answer: Xylazine

93. Name a NSAID and an Antiseptic that can't be used in cats due to toxicity?

Answer: Paracetamol (NSAID) and Cresol (Antiseptic)

94. The first hormone synthesized in the laboratory

Answer: Thyroxine

95. The antidote of coumarine poisoning

Answer: Menadion

96. Posology deals with which part of pharmacology?

Answer: Determination of dosage

97. Name a mycotoxin primarily affects kidney

Answer: Ochratoxin

98. The subacute selenium toxicity is termed as

Answer: Blind Staggers

99. Bitter almond smell and Garlic smell is an indication of which toxicity?

Answer: Cyanide toxicity (Bitter almond smell), Phosphorus toxicity (garlic smell)

100. What is Humane Method of slaughtering?

Answer: Humane slaughtering of animals refers to the practice of killing animals in a way that minimizes pain, suffering, and distress. This can involve methods and practices including stunning the animal prior to slaughter, using precise and sharp equipment to reduce discomfort, creating a serene and comfortable setting, and making sure the animal is handled with respect and dignity throughout the process.

In order to satisfy the demands of the food business and customers, humane slaughter aims to ensure that animals are slaughtered in a way that is as humane and ethical as possible. Species, local laws and regulations, as well as cultural and religious beliefs, can all influence the precise procedures and criteria for humane slaughter.

101. Which bleeding technique is best for quality meat production?

Answer: Thoracic sticking is used to speed up the bleeding process by placing a metal blade into the incision and destroying the jugular vein and carotid artery from the heart. As the majority of the blood drains from the carcass, it is more hygienic.

102. What is Jhatka method of slaughter?

Answer: Jhatka is a particular kind of ritual slaughter that is mostly done in Sikhism and Hinduism. In Jhatka, the animal's head is instantly cut, resulting to slowly bleeding to death. In contrast, here bleeding produces is less than halal. Hence, the meat produced using this method of killing is firm, has a shorter shelf life, but has a higher nutritional content.

103. For quality meat production which slaughtering method is the best?

Answer: Halal method. Since the central nervous system is not severed, the Halal method results in complete blood draining. Consequently, the meat that is produced is soft and has a long shelf life.

104. What is stunning?

Answer: The procedure of putting an animal unconscious or pain-insensitive before being slaughtered is known as stunning.

Several techniques, such as electric shock, captive bolt, gas inhalation, or physical force, are frequently used for stunning. The goal of stunning is to reduce the animal's pain and suffering throughout the slaughter procedure while also improving worker safety and efficiency. When an animal is properly stunned, it will lose consciousness or become pain-insensitive, making the slaughter procedure more compassionate and under control. The type of stunning technique utilized will vary according on the species and size of the animal, regional laws, and industry requirements.

105. Name some stunning methods used on livestock

Answer: In modern slaughterhouses a variety of stunning methods are used on livestock.

a) Electrical stunning (High voltage alternate electric current is sent through brain)

b) Chemical or Gaseous stunning (animals are exposed to a mixture of breathing gases like CO_2, argon, nitrogen *etc.* causing asphyxia)

c) Mechanical or Percussive stunning (a device is used which hits the animal on the skull, with or without penetration leading to immediate unconsciousness by brain trauma. For instance, a captive bolt gun, a water jet stunner, or a pneumatic stunner).

106. In Kosher slaughter method the act of killing is known as

Answer: Shechita

107. What is Halal?

Answer: Islamic ritual slaughtering of livestock or fowl involves severing the jugular vein, carotid artery, and windpipe to cause death. When an animal is killed, it must be conscious and in good health, and the carcass is completely bloodless.

108. For electric stunning which electricity parameter is good for a pig?

Answer: Alternate Current 300 volts for 3 seconds. A minimum of 1.25 - 1.3 amps must be passed through pigs' brain.

109. What are the signs of effective stun by electric stunning method?

Answer: Animal immediately collapses with opisthotonos, rolling of the eyes downward, muscular flaccidity, and clonic tonic spasm transforming into it. We refer to these symptoms as electro lectic fit.

110. What is legging?

Answer: While removing the skin off sheep and goats, the skin is first removed around the leg to expose and release the hock tendon, which is then used to hang the carcass, this process is called legging.

111. What is dressing percentage?

Answer: The percentage of an animal's carcass weight relative to its live weight.

Dressing Percentage= (Carcass weight ÷ live weight) × 100. (Expressed in per cent)

112. What are the main advantages and disadvantages of various stunning techniques?

Answer:

Method	*Advantages*	*Disadvantages*
Electrical Stunning	a. Immediate stun	a. Involves isolation of individual animal b. Involves restraint c. Poorer carcass quality due to splash or burn d. Stunning efficiency may vary with the operator placement of the electrodes or state of the stunning equipment.
Gas Stunning	a. Can be stunned in groups b. Minimal human handling c. Restraint not needed d. Improved carcass quality due to increased blood yield by 0.75 per cent e. Less noise f. No chance of hazard to operator g. Bone fractures and muscular hemorrhages reduced.	a. Does not cause an immediate stun b. Causes pain and distress for brief period. (≈30sec) c. Need more rooms (expensive) d. Good for pigs
Percussive Stunning	a. Good for cattle, sheep, goat	a. Low slaughter rate as the procedure itself is time consuming b. Not suitable for bulls or pigs (thick frontal bone) c. Noise produced too much, that is unpleasant to next animals

113. Name some factors affecting the dressing percentage

Answer: Factors affecting dressing Percentage are:

a. Breed of the animal,
b. Weather condition,
c. Transport before slaughtering,
d. Feeding of the animal,
e. Gut feel,

f. Fatness,
g. Sale method,
h. Slaughtering technique, *i.e.* Bleeding time *etc.*

114. What are the standard dressing percentage of different carcass?

Answer:

Sl.No.	*Animal*		*Dressing Percentage (per cent)*
1	Buffalo		43-54
2	Sheep		40-50
3	Goat		43-52
4	Pig		70-75
5	Poultry	Broiler	70
		Hen	60-65
		Duck	60-65

115. What is offal meat?

Answer: Offal, is a term for a variety of non-muscular animal body parts, such as internal organs and guts, that are either eaten raw or used to prepare other dishes. The liver, lung, heart, and gut, as examples.

Chapter 4

Livestock Production Management

PART A: CATTLE AND BUFFALO

1. **The most distinct external feature between Zebu cattle and European cattle**

   Answer: The presence of a hump in Zebu cattle is the most distinct external feature from that of European cattle.

2. **What are the differences between *Bos indicus* and *Bos taurus*?**

   Answer: *Bos indicus* (Zebu) have generally better heat tolerance, disease resistance (especially tick-borne infections), and a lower basal metabolic rate than *Bos taurus* (European cattle). Zebu cattle look different from its' European counterparts and they have distinct features like hump, long face, drooping ears, upright horn, loose skin, prominent brisket area and dewlap. Zebu cattle also mature late and are comparatively poor milk producers compared to European cattle.

3. **Who is a better converter of crude fiber among cattle and buffalo?**

   Answer: Buffaloes convert poor quality roughage better into high quality animal protein. Buffaloes have around 5 per cent better digestibility of crude fiber than high-yielder cattle.

4. Which category of buffalo produces the majority of milk?

Answer: Buffaloes are classified into two categories: swamp buffalo (2n chromosome= 48) and riverine (2n chromosome= 50) *i.e.*, river or water buffalo. Riverine buffaloes produce about 90 per cent of the total milk coming out of buffaloes; examples of riverine buffaloes are Murraha, Nili Ravi, Mehsana, *etc.*

5. Lactation period

Answer: The length of milk production after calving is known as the lactation period and lactation records are generally expressed on a 305-day basis. For comparison of the milk yield of different animals, the milk yield should be converted to 4 per cent fat-corrected milk.

6. One calf a year

Answer: The target of breeding and reproduction management is to obtain one calf per year in cattle as it is more profitable in terms of milk production, total number of calves obtained per cow and to maintain the reproductive cycle.

7. What is the recommended dry period for cattle?

Answer: The period from the date the milch cow stops milk production to the next calving is considered as the dry period. A dry period of 45-65 days is recommended; a shorter dry period may lead to low milk production in the coming lactation, poor health of the developing fetus and other health issues related to the pregnant cow.

8. Management of a new born calf

Answer:

a) Mucous or membrane adhering to a just-born calf is normally cleaned by the mother cow by licking; if assistance is required, it may be facilitated to remove the same with care.

b) If any problem is seen in normal breathing of the calf, it may be assisted by tickling the nostril, pressing and relaxing the chest wall, or by other suitable methods.

c) The navel cord should be aseptically tied and cut and apply tincture iodine for 3-4 days to prevent any infection.

d) The calf should take colostrum at the earliest possible time, preferrable within 30 minutes, if not then must be within 2 hours. A calf may be assisted in suckling if needed. A calf should take colostrum at the rate of 12-15 per cent of its own body weight.

e) Proper housing and nutrition care for calf should be done. If needed, mineral or vitamin supplements like vitamins A, D, and E may be provided.

The calf starts nibbling at around 14 days of age, so good quality fodder should be kept during this period. If feasible a good quality milk replacer may be provided.

f) Deworming may be done at 21 days and if necessary, earlier. Vaccination can begin as schedules.

9. Milk feeding schedule in calf

Answer: The colostrum should be fed to the calf as soon as possible after calving and be fed for 2-3 days at the rate of 12–15 per cent of calf weight. Then whole milk is fed to calf at the rate of $1/10^{th}$ of the calf's body weight up to 30 days of age; after that, it may be fed at the rate of $1/20^{th}$ of the calf's body weight.

10. What is the difference between milk replacer and calf starter?

Answer: Milk replacer is a prepared feed having nutritional value similar to that of milk that is diluted with water to feed to calves as an economic rearing measure and to save milk from the cow. Calf starter is prepared to provide pre-ruminant calf with high energy and protein. Calf starter contains 75–80 per cent TDN and 16–20 per cent CP, whereas milk replacer contains 20–22 per cent CP and 10–20 per cent crude fat. Milk replacers are costlier and contain skim milk powder (10–15 per cent) and vegetable or animal fat, which is usually not provided in calf starter.

11. What is Calf scour?

Answer: Neonatal diarrhoea is characterized by faeces that are frequently chalky white in colour and have a strong odour. Scour can be due to infective agents, over or quick consumption of milk by the calf, or mechanical reasons like hair balls in the abomasum. Infective origin scour can be treated with antibiotics, and nutritive origin scour can be treated by keeping the calf off feed for 24 hours and providing a limited amount of milk diluted with lukewarm water.

12. What does pot belly and swelling under the jaw signifies in calf?

Answer: Parasite infestation.

13. When should cows in a farm be observed for heat?

Answer: Signs of heat should be observed at least twice daily, *i.e.*, in the morning and evening.

14. What is the best indicator of heat in cattle?

Answer: Standing heat is the best indicator, *i.e.*, standing when mounted by other cows.

15. What is a "marker bull" or "teaser bull"?

Answer: A marker or teaser bull is one of those male animals that have been surgically modified so that they cannot breed cattle in heat but are used for heat detection. Surgical modifications like vasectomy, penis deviation, penectomy, *etc.* are done to prevent the animal from breeding.

16. What is the thumb rule for doing artificial insemination in cattle?

Answer: If a cow shows heat in the morning, it should be bred in the evening, and if it shows heat in the evening, it should be bred the next morning.

17. What do you mean by steaming up in cattle?

Answer: Providing an extra allowance of feed for the impending calving is known as steaming up in cattle. Beginning with 1.5 kg of extra concentrate per day about two months before the calving date and gradually increasing to 4-5 kg per day until the last 2-3 days before parturition. Benefits of steaming include a well-developed foetus, a longer lactation period, and higher milk fat.

18. Which hormone may counteract the effect of oxytocin during milking (if disturbed)?

Answer: Adrenalin

19. Why should milking be completed as soon as possible?

Answer: Milk let-down is controlled by nervous and hormonal action. Oxytocin is the milk let down hormone, which causes muscular contractions around the alveoli and ducts, forcing milk into larger ducts and gland cisterns. The action of oxytocin lasts for 5-7 minutes, so milking must be done within this period to bring out most of the milk from the udder.

20. Lead or challenge feeding

Answer: Lead or challenge feeding is adapted for high yielders, where high levels of concentrate are fed to milch cows to exploit their capacity for maximum milk production. Concentrate feeding is increased by 450–900 g every day for 2–3 weeks, starting three days after calving. The level of concentrate feeding is kept constant at peak milk production, and with a decrease in production, the level of concentrate feeding is decreased.

21. What is the principle of machine milking?

Answer: The principle of machine milking is to apply negative and atmospheric pressure through a double-chambered teat cup, thus creating a pressure difference across the teat canal by applying vacuum to the teat end to extract milk.

A Pulsation of 45-60 times per minute is usually maintained.

22. **Which exotic breed of cattle produces the highest milk fat percent?**

Answer: Jersey (4.5 per cent fat and even higher).

23. **Low roughage, high concentrate diet reduces the fat content of milk.**

Answer: Cattle digest fiber due to the action of microbial fermentation, and dietary fiber improves milk fat percentage by increasing the amount of acetate, which is a precursor for the synthesis of milk fat. As a result, low roughage will result in lower acetate and, as a result, a lower milk fat percentage.

24. **Is milking 3 to 4 times done in high yielding cattle?**

Answer: In very high yielders, milking three times a day increases the production of milk by 10–25 per cent compared to milking twice a day, and milking four times a day increases production by 5–15 per cent compared to milking three times a day. Often, in high-yield cows, milking is done three times, but four times milking is generally not practiced as it is often not feasible or economically viable.

25. **Does milker efficiency affect fat and SNF percentage?**

Answer: Yes. Milking is a specialized job, and the efficiency of the milker certainly affects the total fat and SNF percent in the milk produced by hand milking.

26. **What are the drying off methods?**

Answer: Methods of drying off 1. Sudden cessation of milking 2. Intermittent milking; and 3. Incomplete milking. Sudden cessation of milking leads to pressure building up, which leads to regression of milk secretory cells. This method is suitable for low yielders. In high yielders incomplete milking is practiced, where the cows are milked gradually in smaller quantities. In the intermittent milking procedure, cows are milked intermittently every second or third day until milk production ceases entirely.

27. **What precautions should be taken in drying off?**

Answer: A proper method of drying off should be followed, taking into consideration the milk production of the dairy cattle. 2. Proper teat sealing with appropriate antibiotics may be done to prevent the occurrence of mastitis. 3. The udder should be checked for 2–3 weeks post-drying for any swelling or abnormalities.

28. **What are steps to be followed for clean milk production?**

Answer: Education and training of milk producers in proper hygiene, housekeeping, sanitation, milking techniques, and animal husbandry procedures should be the first step towards clean milk production. The various strategies for clean milk production may be as follows:

a) Training and awareness of farmers, workers *etc.*
b) Proper nutrition and feeding of animals.
c) Housing management including cleaning, sanitation and disinfection of animal houses.
d) Proper milking vessels and there scientific handling is needed. Small topped stainless-steel utensils, regularly cleaned following standard protocol is needed to maintain clean milk production.
e) Health management of milch animals and udder hygiene should be followed. Regular health monitoring of animals for diseases like mastitis, tuberculosis *etc.*, should be done. Proper teat dipping, washing of udder, udder clipping *etc.*, should be followed. Pre-dipping is highly effective to control mastitis.
f) Cleanliness and health of milkers is important, especially they should be free from contagious diseases like tuberculosis, typhoid, cholera *etc.*
g) Scientific milk collection and transportation is a must for clean milk production. Milk is highly perishable item and good media for growth of microbes, so proper collection, early cooling to around 4°C and early transportation is important.

29. Care and management of breeding bulls

Answer:

a) Properly balanced nutrition should be provided with supplementation of vitamins like A, D, E, and selenium and minerals during breeding season to maintain fertility. Extra allowances of concentrate and leguminous fodder may be provided during breeding season as and when required. The bulls should neither be too lean nor too fat.
b) Separate housing should be provided to bulls with adequate prescribed space and facilities. A breeding bull should receive plenty of exercise for proper body condition and fertility.
c) Bulls should be handled properly as they are generally aggressive. Bull rings may be used as they are easier to control.
d) Proper grooming, cleaning, and washing are needed to maintain the bull's condition.
e) Regular evaluation of health status and screening for certain diseases should be done. Regular deworming and vaccinations should be followed. From time to time, semen screening should be done to assess the fertility of the animal.

30. What is the draught power of a bullock?

Answer: The power developed by a bull in horse power (HP) is known as draught power. Bullocks generally produce draught equivalent to 1/5–1/6th of their body weight, which is 0.74 HP. The buffalo generates 0.75 HP and the cow 0.45 HP.

31. Calfhood vaccination

Answer: Vaccination against brucella is only done in female calves between the ages of 4 and 8 months, also known as childhood vaccination, using a brucella cotton 19 strain vaccine.

Currently, a brucella control program is being implemented throughout the country to control this highly important zoonotic disease.

32. What schedule should be followed for deworming cattle? Can we treat cattle with anthelmintics during pregnancy?

Answer: The first deworming may be done at 21 days to 1 month of calf age. Up to 6 months of age, deworm every month, then 2 times annually (stall fed animals) to 4 times (grazaing animal) or as and when required. It is always advocated to deworm animals before and after the rainy season, as the parasitic load would be highest during this period. Deworming two weeks before vaccination is advisable, as it ensures the efficacy of the vaccine. Deworming is done based on the weight of the individual animal, and it is good to regularly change the group of dewormers.

If there is any need for anthelmintics during the pregnancy period, they can be used; certain groups of anthelmintics have no such adverse effect on pregnancy.

33. What managemental practices can be followed to prevent mastitis?

Answer:

a) Proper nutrition to maintain udder health is the foremost. Essential vitamins and minerals may also be supplemented as and when required to maintain udder health.

b) Care and hygiene of the udder and teats. Using teat dips or pre-dipping is a very effective way to prevent mastitis. 3/4th of the surface of the teat should be covered by pre-dips, and there should be a contact time of at least 30 seconds.

c) Maintaining the cleanliness and hygiene of milkers and milking machines is important. Regular washing/disinfection of hands in the case of hand milking should be followed to prevent the spread of infection from one animal to another.

d) Regular cleaning and disinfection of animal houses should be done. Dry and clean floors are ideal.

e) Do not allow cattle to lie down immediately after milking. Feeding greens after milking can be a good option to keep them standing for 30–40 minutes, and in the meantime, the dilated opening of the teats would return to normal, preventing the entry of harmful pathogens from the floor while lying down.

f) Regular screening of milk and screening of pooled milk should be done for early detection and treatment. A Californian mastitis test should be done immediately for any suspected case for confirmation.

g) Special care should be taken during drying off, and teats should be properly sealed in the case of high yielders with standard formulations available in the market. During the transition phase, *i.e.*, 3 weeks before and 3 weeks after calving, proper care and observation are a must, as this is the most critical phase.

34. Anthrax vaccine is provided only in the endemic zone or in areas where there is any out break

Answer: Anthrax is a zoonotic disease of high importance and its vaccination is done only in the endemic zone or in areas where there is an outbreak.

35. What should be the culling rate in an organized farm?

Answer: The culling rate should ideally be less than 20 per cent in an organized farm.

36. When judging a dairy cow, which trait has the highest number on the scorecard?

Answer: Udder, having a maximum number or score of 40. Udder scoring depends on udder depth, rear udder, fore udder, teat placement, udder balance, texture, *etc.*

37. What is Freemartin?

Answer: When twin calves of different sexes are born, the male calf is sexually normal but the female calf is usually sterile and the external genitalia are abnormal; such females are known as freemartins.

38. The most common and convenient method of controlling adult cattle and buffalo in veterinary centers

Answer: Using trevis or crush

39. Common method to cast cattle on the ground

Answer: Reuff's method and Burley's method.

40. How can you determine the age of cattle in field conditions if you have no records?

Answer: By examining the dentition of the animal.

41. Which breed of cattle is native to West Bengal?

Answer: Siri is found in the hilly tracts of Darjeeling.

42. **Which one is the best dual-purpose breed of cattle in India?**

Answer: Hariana

43. **What is the cattle and buffalo breeding policy of West Bengal?**

Answer: Cattle and buffalo breeding policy for West Bengal (2007)

a) Only non-descript animals in the state will be upgraded with improved indigenous breed. The Sahiwal and Gir breeds will be used for upgradation.

b) In the districts of Alipurduar, Kalimpong, Darjeeling, Coochbehar, Jalpaiguri, Uttar Dinajpur, Dakshin Dinajpur, Malda, Murshidabad, Nadia, and Hooghly,Purba Bardhaman, Purba Medinipur, Paschim medinipur and Howrah, Sahiwal breed will be employed. Gir breed will be used in North 24-Parganas, South 24-Parganas, Birbhum, Purulia, Bankura, Paschim Bardhaman and Jhargram. The farmer's preference will be taken into consideration when deciding which of the two descript breeds to adopt for improvement in any of the aforementioned zones.

c) Upgradation and cross-breeding will be 80 per cent and 20 per cent, respectively, of the total cattle population.

d) For the purpose of Cross-breeding, only Jersey will be used for its smaller size and improved adaptability to the agro-climatic environment of West Bengal.

e) The crossing of existing crossbreeds may be done in a restricted manner and the exotic inheritance shall not be increased beyond 50 per cent. Semen of Holstein Friesian or its crosses, may be provided by the Paschim Banga Go-Sampad Bikash Sanstha (PBGSBS) to farmers interested in rearing Holstein crossbreeds with proper application.

f) The grading-up with high quality Murrah Buffalo semen in all parts of the state should be followed for buffaloes.

44. **Which breed of buffalo produces the highest milk fat percent?**

Answer: Bhadawari Buffalo (14 per cent milk fat)

45. **What are the various grazing systems?**

Answer: The various grazing systems are controlled continuous grazing, deferred grazing, rotational grazing, rotational deferred grazing and Hohenheim system of grazing.

46. **The mainstay of AMUL dairy in the Anand district**

Answer: Surti Buffalo

47. **How many liters of blood pass through the udder for the synthesis of 1 liter of milk?**

Answer: 500 liters.

48. Persistency of lactation

Answer: The degree of maintenance of milk production or the rate of decline in milk yield after peak yield is measured in ratios of yield, by variations in yield, or through model parameters.

49. Why milking is called as labour-intensive operation?

Answer: Hand milking requires 50-60 per cent of the total man hours spent in a dairy farm.

50. Best method of selection

Answer: The selection index method is the best method of selection, where each character, depending on its heritability and economic importance, is assigned a value, and on the basis of these values, the animal is given a score.

PART B: GOAT

1. "Poor man's cow" or "wet nurse" of infants

Answer: Goat

2. Best goat meat (Chevon) breed

Answer: Black Bengal goats. Also known for its high-quality leather.

3. Mohair

Answer: Goat hair obtained from Angora goats.

4. Pashmina (cashmere of fine quality)

Answer: Fine quality downy coats or winter undercoats are obtained from Chegu and Changthangi goats.

5. Scientific name of goat

Answer: *Capra hircus*

6. High milk yielding exotic breeds of goat

Answer: Saanen, Toggenburg, Alpine, and Nubian.

7. Gestation period of goat?

Answer: 150 days

8. The unique feeding behavior of goat is different from other species

Answer: Browsing habit and is often known as a bipedal feeder.

9. Popular identification methods in goats.

Answer: Ear tags, neck tags, and tattooing.

10. What is the importance of castration in goats?

Answer: Importance of castration are

a) Castration leads to higher meat production and improves the quality of meat produced.

b) Prevent goaty odour in meat

c) Makes the animal docile

11. Common methods of castration in goats at field level

Answer:

a) The bloodless method by Burdizzo's castrator (most preferred).

b) Open surgery method

11. Name the probable first ruminant to be domesticated.

Answer: Probably goats were the first ruminant and animal after dog to be domesticated at about 9000-7000 BC (Neolithic age).

12. What is special about goat milk?

Answer: Goat milk is wholesome, nutritious, easily digestible (smaller fat globules), and closest to human milk. Goat milk being alkaline is often recommended in different diseased conditions like peptic ulcer, jaundice *etc.* The average fat globule size in goat milk is 3.5μm which allows for better homogenized milk fat and digestibility. Higher levels of short and medium chain fatty acids allow for the treatment of a variety of fat malabsorption syndromes. Goat milk contains 10 times more oligosaccharides than cow milk.

13. Goats are prone to which disease?

Answer: Broncho-pneumonia

14. What do you mean by "tethering" in goat farming?

Answer: Tethering is a form of semi-intensive goat farming where goats are tied to a peg or fence line or tree with a rope (3-5 meters long). The length of the rope represents the available grazing area for the goat and by regular shifting of the peg/post a new grazing area is provided.

15. Name some fiber purpose goats.

Answer: Gaddi, Marwari, Chegu, and Changthangi.

16. What type of housing will be comfortable for goats?

Answer: Goats do not require elaborate housing but it should be well ventilated with proper drainage. The house should get sufficient light and they prefer dry, safe and comfortable housing. Slatted floors are often used in housing, as goats have special liking for dry floors.

17. What is the dry matter intake in goats?

Answer: Meat type goats take around 3 per cent of their live weight in dry matter, while milch or dairy goats have a higher requirement of around 4-5 per cent.

18. What do you mean by "zero grazing feeding system" in goats?

Answer: Also known as stall feeding, where goats are confined in stalls and are not allowed to graze, this practice is generally followed in cities or in areas where grazing pasture availability is low or non-existent.

19. How much colostrum feeding is advisable for goat kids?

Answer: Colostrum equal to 10 per cent of body weight within 24 hours of birth.

20. Kids are weaned at what age in goat farming?

Answer: At any time up to 6 months age, but it is more scientific to wean within 3 months of age of the kids.

21. Based on rearing practices, which types of goats will have better muscle to bone ratio?

Answer: Goats raised on intensive and semi-intensive systems have a better muscle to bone ratio than goats reared on an extensive system.

22. Dressing percentage in goats?

Answer: 45-55 per cent

23. Name a heavy indigenous goat breed.

Answer: Jamunapari

24. What would be the average weight of a Black Bengal goat?

Answer: Black Bengal goats are a light weight breed; adult males weigh around 14-15 kg and adult females around 8-13 kg.

25. What is the coat colour of a Bengal goat?

Answer: Predominantly black, though grey, white and brown are also found

26. Bucks of what age should be used for breeding?

Answer: 18-24 months

27. Optimum ratio of buck to Doe

Answer: 1:40-50

28. Which is the most prolific domestic ruminant?

Answer: Goat

29. What is the average birth weight of a Black Bengal kid?

Answer: 1.1-1.2 Kg

30. Age at puberty in a goat

Answer: 5-7 months

31. Is artificial insemination successful in goats?

Answer: Yes

32. Name some good milk producing Indian breeds of goat.

Answer: Beetal, Jamunapari, Barbari, Malabari *etc.*

33. Name the common diseases of goats.

Answer: PPR (*Peste des Petes Ruminants*), CCPP (Contagious Caprine Pleura-pneumonia), Enterotoxaemia, Goat Pox, FMD (Foot and Mouth Disease), Brucella, Coccidia, Contagious Ecthyma, Mastitis, Endo-parasitic, Ecto-parasitic *etc.*

34. What leads to the typical goaty flavour in chevo?

Answer: 4-methyloctanoic fatty acid (hircinoic acid).

35. Goat manure

Answer: It contains a higher amount of nitrogen (2.04 per cent) and phosphorus (0.73 per cent) than cattle or buffalo manure.

36. Which goat breed have parrot mouth appearance?

Answer: Jamunapari have Roman nose with a tuft of hair, giving them a parrot mouth appearance.

37. Which indigenous goat breeds produce triplets and quadruplets?

Answer: Black Bengal and Barbari. Black Bengal goats kids twice a year, Barbari twice in 14-16 months and other breeds generally kids three times in two years.

38. Name the goat breeds that are considered threatened?

Answer: Chegu, Surti, Jamunapari and to some extent Beetal.

39. How much space is required by an adult goat?

Answer: 1.25-1.5 square meter.

40. Is goat rearing advocated in ecologically fragile zones?

Answer: Goats do not pose such a threat to ecology as previously assumed, so goat farming can be done in ecologically fragile zones.

PART C: SHEEP

1. Sheep are reared for

Answer: Sheep are mainly reared for meat, wool, skin, manure and to some extent milk and carrying loads.

2. Scientific name of sheep

Answer: *Ovies aries*

3. Fat tailed sheep of India

Answer: Bhakarwal

4. In India, sheep are primarily reared for

Answer: Meat and secondarily for fine and carpet wool.

5. "Mortgage lifter" and golden hoofed animal

Answer: Sheep

6. Why are sheep considered hardy animals?

Answer: Sheep can survive on sparse vegetation as they are inherently strong and have a cleft in their upper lip, which allows very close grazing. Don't require elaborate housing and can be kept even in the open. Sheep are less affected by extreme weather and can resist drought and semi-starvation. The woolly body coat of sheep protects the sheep from rain, hot sun, and abrasions, and they are also less susceptible to diseases.

7. What do you mean by "sheep folding"?

Answer: The penning of sheep in agricultural fields that have been harvested is known as sheep folding. This is practiced to improve the fertility of the soil as sheep penned on a particular field will defecate and urinate and their manure has a high fertilizer value which acts as farmyard manure.

8. Central Sheep and Wool Research Institute (CSWRI)

Answer: Located at Avikanagar, Rajasthan

9. A sheep flock follows its leader sheep and this is aided by

Answer: Pheromones are released by foot gland in the hind foot of sheep.

10. How do goat and sheep feeding behaviour differ?

Answer: Sheep are close grazers and less selective in feeding. Whereas goats are browsers and more selective in feeding. Goats also prefer more variety in feed and have a higher sense of taste than sheep. Browsing tree leaves is in the behaviour of goats, which is contrary to sheep.

11. What do you mean by flushing in sheep?

Answer: Flushing refers to providing ewes with higher nutrition starting about 2 weeks before the start of breeding season so that there is higher ovulation, fertilization, and lambing (5–10 per cent minimum). Flushing also provides other benefits like synchronization of oestrus and building up the body's reserves for a developing foetus and impending lactation.

12. Gestation period of sheep

Answer: Average 147 days (142-152 days).

13. Flock mating in sheep

Answer: In this mating system, males are allowed to run along with females throughout the day and night.

14. What are the commonly occurring diseases in sheep?

Answer: Blue tongue, Anthrax, FMD, Black quarter, HS, Ecto-parasites and endo-parasites *etc.*

15. Dressing percentage of sheep meat (mutton)

Answer: 40-50 per cent

16. What are the properties on which the quality of wool depends?

Answer: Staple length, spinning quality, soundness, elasticity, softness, felting property, trueness, *etc.*

17. How is wool sheared in India?

Answer: The process of completely removing wool is known as shearing. Shearing is done mainly by hand in India, and other methods include hand machine and power machine shearing. The chemical shearing method (injected cyclophosphamide at 24 mg/kg body weight) is also available but not in practice in India.

18. What are the wool grading systems?

Answer: British system, *i.e.*, the spinning count system, and the American or blood system

19. What category of wool is mainly produced in India?

Answer: Coarse type Carpet wool

20. How would you differentiate between wool and hair?

Answer:

Wool	*Hair*
Medulla is almost absent.	Medulla Present
Thickness less	More thickness
Fiber is soft.	Fiber is less soft.
Retains more heat.	Retains relatively less heat.
Permanent dyeing property	Temporary dyeing property

21. Pelt

Answer: Pelt is the skin of sheep including wool.

22. Stag

Answer: A male sheep castrated after it has attained full secondary sexual characteristics.

23. Seggy

Answer: Ram castrated after the first service.

24. A broken mouthed ewe due to its excellent performance retained in the breeding flock beyond the normal time.

Answer: Crone

25. Sheep with high fecundity

Answer: Garole sheep from the Sundarban area of West Bengal have the FecB Booroola gene.

26. Name some new evolved breeds of sheep in India.

Answer: Kashmir Merino, Hissardale, Avivastra, Avikalin, Bharat Merino and Nilgiri.

27. Apparel wool breeds

Answer: Hissardale, Nilgiri, Kashmir Merino, Avivastra and Nilgiri Sythetics.

28. Carpet wool breeds

Answer: Chokla, Gaddi, Avikalin *etc.*

29. Fine exotic wool breeds of sheep

Answer: Merino, Rambouillet and Polworth.

30. Exotic mutton breeds of sheep

Answer: Suffolk, Dorset, Southdown *etc.*

31. Pelt breed of sheep

Answer: Karakul

32. One of the best indigenous mutton breeds

Answer: Nellore and Mandya

33. Telescoping

Answer: Telescoping is done by introducing a ram into a flock of sheep after keeping it away from them for 2-3 months, which leads to heat in the ewes (70- 80 per cent) in the first oestrus cycle.

34. Merino wool

Answer: Merino and their derivatives produces the finest apparel wool variety which accounts for 40 per cent of the total world's wool production. Average fiber diameter is 18-24μ and spinning count of 64-80s.

35. What is the name of the first cloned sheep?

Answer: The first cloned sheep was named Dolly and was created by the electrofusion of a diploid nucleus from the udder cell of an adult ewe.

PART D: POULTRY

1. What do you mean by the word "poultry"

Answer: The word "poultry" indicates all domesticated species of birds like chickens, ducks, turkeys, Japanese quail, guinea fowl, geese, pigeons, ostriches, emu *etc.*, that are reared for meat, eggs or other poultry products.

2. The study of birds that are not classified as poultry

Answer: Ornithology

3. The scientific or zoological name of poultry birds along with their chromosome numbers

Answer:

Common Name	*Scientific Name*	*Chromosome Number (2n)*
Chicken	*Gallus gallus domesticus*	78
Duck	Anas Platyrynchos	80
Turkey	*Meleagris gallopavo*	80
Goose	*Anser anser*	80

Common Name	*Scientific Name*	*Chromosome Number (2n)*
Japanese quail	*Coturnix coturnix japonica*	78
Guinea fowl	*Numida meleagris*	78
Ostrich	*Struthio camelus*	80
Pigeon	*Columba livia*	80
Muscovy Duck	*Cairina moschata*	80
Emu	*Dromaius novaehollandiae*	82

4. How can we distinguish between male and female chickens by external observation?

Answer: Male chickens (cocks) will have prominently developed spurs, sickle feathers, a larger comb and wattle, pointed, larger heckle feathers (neck area), and papillae (rudimentary penis) in comparison to female (hen) chickens. In addition, females have a roundish body, and the feathering pattern and colour may also vary based on breed specifications.

5. What is the unique feature of poultry in terms of its bones?

Answer: Pneumatic bones. These types of bones are light which allows birds to have easy flight and better efficiency in respiration.

6. What do you mean by birds are uricotelic? What is vent/cloaca?

Answer: Birds are uricotelic; the end product of nitrogen metabolism is uric acid and they release their waste products in the form of uric acid.

The vent/cloaca is the common opening for excretion and reproduction/egg laying in poultry birds.

7. What is preen gland?

Answer: The uropygial gland in ducks and waterfowl, found at the back at the base of the tail, is also known as the preen gland. The oil secreted acts as a lubricant and protector for the feathers and skin in these birds.

8. How much water is required for duck farming?

Answer: Ducks need to immerse or wash their heads; otherwise, their eyes become scaly and crusty, which may lead to blindness in extreme cases. So, tubs or water arrangements deep and wide enough to dip the duck heads are good enough for duck farming. Ducks also choose to wash their bills regularly, but extensive water bodies like ponds, rivers, *etc.* for swimming can be a disadvantage in terms of egg and meat production.

9. What are the unique features of a duck?

Answer: Ducks, on external observation, look unique in terms of webbed (palmate) feet, having a bill, and having a bigger and plumper body. Ducks generally can lay up to 2-3 years of age, are comparatively more resistant to the majority of chicken diseases, and lay larger eggs (70-80 g) than chickens. Ducks have a higher requirement for water and require water to dip their heads frequently.

10. Which poultry species has snood and caruncles?

Answer: Turkey

11. In which species of poultry are females larger than males?

Answer: Japanese Quail

12. Can we rear any type of quail for economic purposes?

Answer: No. Only domesticated Japanese Quail can be raised as farm birds for economic reasons. Wild quail or native quail birds are restricted by the Wild Life Protection Act of 1972.

13. What is the average weight and incubation period of common poultry bird eggs?

Answer:

Species	*Egg Weight*	*Incubation Period (Days)*
Ostrich	1200-1500g	42
Duck	70-75g	28
Turkey	80-85g	28
Chicken	50-60g	21
Quail	10-12 g	17-18

14. Classification of chicken

Answer: Based on the place of origin or utility of birds. Based on the origin of birds, the following classification is as follows:

Type (Place of origin)	*Example*
Asiatic	Brahma, Langshan, Cochin *etc.*
American	Plymouth Rock, Rhode Island Red, Wyandotte *etc.*
Mediterranean	Leghorn, Minorca, Ancona *etc.*
English	Orpington, Sussex, Cornish, Australorp *etc.*

Based on utility	
Utility	*Example*
Egg type	Leghorn, Minorca, Ancona *etc.*
Meat type	Cornish, Brahma, Cochin *etc.*
Dual purpose	RIR, Plymouth Rock, Dorking *etc.*
Fancy type	Polish, Hamburg *etc.*
Game	Aseel *etc.*

15. The true stomach of poultry

Answer: Pro-ventriculus (Glandular stomach)

16. What is the function of gizzard in poultry?

Answer: The gizzard (muscular stomach) is where grinding of feed occurs (particle size reduction), regulation of feed flow occurs, and it responds rapidly to changes in the coarseness of the diet.

17. Function of the Bursa of Fabricius (Cloacal Bursa)

Answer: It is involved in immune function and projects dorsally from the proctodeum.

18. Is feeding grits always important when commercially prepared feeds are fed to poultry?

Answer: The presence of grit is not a necessity when commercially prepared feeds are fed, as the feed-grinding process adequately reduces the size of ingredients, thus facilitating gizzard activity.

19. How does a developing avian embryo get energy from an egg?

Answer: The energy requirements of avian embryos during incubation are fulfilled by lipids stored in the yolk.

20. Recognized breeds of duck in India

Answer: Pati (Assam) and Maithili (Bihar).

21. Some breeds of ducks found in India which have not been recognized yet by the NBAGR

Answer: Sythetmet, Nageswari ducks of the North Eastern states, Kuttanad ducks of Kerala (varieties Chara and Chemballi), and Arani ducks of Tamil Nadu.

22. Only recognised poultry breed from West Bengal

Answer: Harringhata Black

23. Name the recognised (NBAGR) chicken breeds of India.

Answer: Aseel (known for its fighting ability), Busra, Chittagong, Danki, Deothigir, Ghagus, Hansli, Hasringhata Balck, Kadaknath, Kalasthi, Kashmir Fevorolla, Kaunayen, Mewari, Miri, Nicobari, Punjab Brown, Tellichery, Uttara, and Ankaleshwar.

24. Characteristics of the Kadaknath breed of poultry.

Answer: The breeding tract is Madhya Pradesh (some districts of Rajasthan and Gujarat also), with day-old chicks having characteristic bluish to black colour and irregular dark stripes over the back. In adults, the comb, wattles, and tongue are purple. The shining blue tinge of the ear lobes adds to its unique features. Most of the internal organs show characteristic black pigmentation, and the black colour is due to melanin pigment. (Fibro melanosis). Mainly used for meat and socio-cultural and religious ceremonies. Meat is considered to have medicinal value and fetches a high price.

25. Ancestor of the chicken

Answer: Red Jungle fowl

26. What are LIT birds?

Answer: Low Input Technology birds. ICAR and the Government of India have been working on developing birds that look like native chickens and suit rural production systems. They are characterized by being multi-coloured and are camouflaged from predators. It lays a considerable number of eggs, has a faster growth rate than native chickens, can sustain itself on a low quantity of feed, and can survive under scavenging. Examples of LIT birds are Vanaraja, Gramapriya, Krishi-bro, Kuroiler, Hitacari, Upakari, *etc.*

27. What type of chicken breeds are generally distributed in government schemes for backyard poultry?

Answer: For backyard poultry, indigenous and LIT birds are generally preferred, though dual-purpose breeds like RIR are also distributed in various government schemes. Generally, no high-producing commercial breeds or strains are provided as they require high inputs in terms of feeding, housing, and management, which are difficult to provide in backyard poultry farming by resource-poor farmers. Moreover, the agility, camouflage ability, and capacity to escape from predators of commercial strains in backyard farming are not up to the mark.

28. Generally, which ovary is active in poultry?

Answer: Left ovary

29. What do you mean by table egg?

Answer: An unfertilized egg is table egg.

30. Where does the colour of the yolk come from:

Answer: The colour of the yolk comes from fat-soluble pigments called xanthophylls contained in the hen's diet. Birds fed diets with yellow maize or allowed to range on grass typically produce eggs with deep yellow yolks.

31. Different parts of chicken oviduct and its functions.

Answer:

Segment	*Function*	*Time spent*
Infundibulum	Yolk is picked up by the ovum.	15 minutes
Magnum	Albumen	3 hours
Isthmus	Inner and outer shell membrane	75 minutes
Uterus	Water and salts are added through the shell membrane. Egg shell calcification.	18-20 hours
Vagina	Cuticle deposited on shell pores	Few minutes

32. What is the time required by a chicken (hen) to produce an egg?

Answer: The total time a hen's body takes to convert a yolk into a fully developed egg and lay that egg is about 25–26 hours. Generally, after about 30 to 75 minutes after a hen lays an egg, the ovary releases the next ovum.

33. How frequently is artificial insemination done in poultry?

Answer: Near the junction of the shell gland and the vagina are deep glands known as sperm host glands that can store sperm for long periods of time, typically 10 days to 2 weeks. (One of the unique things about birds is that the sperm remain viable at body temperature.) When a hen lays an egg, sperm can be squeezed out of these glands into the oviduct, where from it can migrate to the infundibulum to fertilize an ovum. So, generally 2 times artificial insemination in a week is good enough to maintain the fertility.

34. What is caponization?

Answer: Castration or removal of the testes in roosters (male poultry birds) is referred to as caponization.

35. Testes in chicken males are located

Answer: Inside the body cavity

36. A shell of an egg is composed of

Answer: Calcium carbonate (94 per cent), magnesium carbonate (1 per cent), calcium phosphate (1 per cent) and organic matter (chiefly protein, 4 per cent).

37. Eggs are deficient in which vitamin?

Answer: Vitamin C

38. Is an egg too rich in cholesterol for human consumption?

Answer: A standard chicken egg of 58 grams contains only 258 mg of cholesterol, whereas about 1800–2000 mg of cholesterol is utilized daily by the human body. So, an adult normal human being can take eggs daily without any adverse effects.

39. The shell colour of the egg is very characteristic of the breeds of poultry; how does it affect the quality of the egg?

Answer: The colour of an egg's shell has nothing to do with its quality.

40. How would you differentiate between a good and poor layer?

Answer: Good layers are healthy, vigorous, tight and close feathered, with a large and glossy comb and wattles. Good layers have soft, flexible, well spread pubic bones (2–3 fingers), and soft, thin, and loose skin. The vent in good layers is large, oval, dilated, and moist.

41. At what age do Japanese quail mature?

Answer: At around 5-6 weeks both meat and egg type Japanese quails do mature.

42. Name the highest egg producing duck?

Answer: The Khaki Campbell duck is the highest egg producing duck, developed by Mrs. Campbell in England during the beginning of the 19th century by crossing strains of Fawn, Mallard, Rouen with Indian Runner (White)

43. Which duck has a typical soda water bottle structure?

Answer: Indian Runner duck which are excellent layers.

44. Name few meats type ducks

Answer: White Pekin, Aylesbury, Rouen and Muscovy *etc.*

45. Name a few hybrid ducks.

Answer: Vigova Super-M (broiler duck), Cherry Valley (Dual purpose), Hytop (mule duck) and Legarth (meat-type)

46. The majority of ducks lay by what time of the day?

Answer: 9 A.M. in the morning

47. Name some breeds of geese.

Answer: Toulose, Emden and Roman

48. Most important vaccines for duck

Answer:

Name of Vaccine	*Dose*	*Route*	*Age of vaccination*
Duck Cholera	1 ml	Subcutaneous	3-4 weeks, adults 2 ml after 1 month of their last vaccination or 18 weeks of age.
Duck Plague	1 ml	Subcutaneous	8-12 weeks

49. Does domestic turkey have many breeds?

Answer: Turkeys originated from Northern and Central America and are raised mainly for meat. The domestic turkey belongs to only one breed with a number of varieties. Example: Broad Breasted Bronze, Broad Breasted White, Beltsville White, White Holland, Narragansett, *etc.*

50. Varieties of Guinea fowl

Answer: Pearl, White, Black and Lavender

51. What is the status of poultry farming in India?

Answer: Poultry farming has advanced a lot and is more commonly referred to as the "poultry industry," and a high input/high output production approach is in practice. It is commercial and industrial in nature. The poultry industry in India ranks third in egg production and fifth in meat production. More than fifty percent of the total meat consumed in India comes from poultry. The annual growth rate varies from 8–10 per cent and is one of the fastest growing sectors. In spite of such huge growth, there is tremendous potential for expansion and advancement in the coming decades. The poultry industry has the potential to narrow the protein gap in the diet of such a huge population and also generate employment.

52. What are the advantages of poultry farming?

Answer: Poultry farming has many inherent advantages, including

a) Comparatively initial investment is low.

b) Provides quick/rapid return.

c) Converts feed to good quality protein in very short period of time.

d) Have the potential to generate employment.

e) Relatively less space is required for farming.

f) Poultry waste/manure can be used as fertilizer.

g) Changing food habits and urbanization leading to high demands of animal protein.

53. How many eggs does a commercial chicken layer produce?

Answer: Commercial chicken layer produces 310–320 eggs annually, *i.e.*, around 18 kg of eggs.

54. Physiological zero of egg

Answer: The temperature below which the embryonic growth ceases is known as physiological zero and it is 24° C (75.2° Fl) for chicken egg.

55. At what age is a broiler chicken marketed?

Answer: Generally, at 36–42 days of age, with an average weight of around 2–2.2 kg per bird.

56. Which states in India are the highest poultry egg and meat producers?

Answer: Andhra Pradesh, Tamil Nadu, Telangana, West Bengal, and Haryana are among the top egg producing states in the country, cumulatively contributing about 65 per cent of the total egg production. Maharashtra, Haryana, West Bengal and Tamil Nadu are the leading chicken broiler meat producing states in the country.

57. What is brooding management in chicks?

Answer: The care and management of day-old chicks during the early part of their lives (generally up to 4-6 weeks of age or until they are well feathered) is known as brooding. Chicks require extra heat at this stage due to their poorly developed thermoregulatory mechanism and it takes about two weeks to develop this mechanism and achieve homeostasis. There are generally two types of brooding, *i.e.*, natural brooding (desi broody hens brooding 10–15 chicks/hen) and artificial brooding (practiced in commercial rearing where an artificial heat source is used to maintain temperature).

58. What are the basic requirements of brooding in chicks?

Answer: The basic requirements for brooding in chickens are:

a) Temperature: The optimal brooding temperature during the first week is 90–95°F, and subsequently, the temperature may be reduced at a rate of 5°F on every successive week, until the room temperature of 60–70°F is reached or the chicks are fully feathered.

b) Ventilation: Proper ventilation is necessary to provide fresh air by removing obnoxious gases like CO2, CO, NH3, *etc.*

c) Humidity: About 50–60 per cent relative humidity is sufficient for floor brooding.

d) Feeding Space: Each chick should get a minimum of 2 inches of linear feeding space up to 2-3 weeks and then increase as required/standards, 3 inches up to 6 weeks, and 4 inches up to 12 weeks of age.

e) Watering space: Waterer at regular interval with adequate space should be provided.

f) Floor space: In the brooder house 0.3 sq. ft space per chick is required and avoid placing more than 500 chicks under one brooder.

g) Lighting: 24 hours light is required up to 4-5 days depending upon season, though 1-hour dark period may be provided.

59. Name the best layer and best meat-type chicken breeds.

Answer: Leghorn is the best egg producer, and Cornish is the best meat breed.

60. What are the commonly used brooders in poultry houses?

Answer: Electric lamp brooders, infrared lamps, gas brooders, *etc.*

61. What are the objectives of brooding poultry?

Answer: Brooding is necessary to provide proper care for the young chicks. The objectives of brooding chicks are:

a) To safeguard that chick, grow strong from day-old to 7 days or more of age.

b) To increase appetite and encourage the growth of feathers.

c) To achieve proper target body weight by 2 weeks of age and maintain a smooth growth curve from one day old to 4 weeks of age.

d) To ensure consistency throughout the flock.

65. How to distinguish male and female day-old chicks? Which of the parents' gametes determines the sex of a hatchling in poultry?

Answer: The various methods to determine the sex of day-old chicks include methods involved by using proctoscope, Vent sexing or Japanese method of sexing and in some breeds by feather sexing method (by observation of feather colour).

Females in poultry are classified as ZW because they are heterogametic whereas males are designated as ZZ because they are homogametic. So, a female or hen determines the sex of a hatchling in poultry.

66. How are commercial poultry breeds or strains developed?

Answer: More than 90 per cent of commercial birds are crosses of one kind or another, *i.e.*, strain crosses, breed crosses, and inbred hybrids. Performance in the progeny is enhanced as a result of the crossing. One line is employed as a male line (sire line) and the other as a female line (dam line) to obtain commercial crosses. For the development of commercial chicks, sire and dam lines are those that provide male and female parents. When commercial chicken is a single cross, each line entering the cross is called a parent line. When four lines are used, each line is called a grandparent line.

67. Commercial layers and broiler chickens

Answer: Commercial layers are strains of cross- or inbred hybrids of White Leghorn origin used for the production of white shelled eggs. Whereas crossbreeding White Leghorn as the male parent and RIR, New Hampshire, or Black Australorp as the female parent is used for the production of commercial layers for tinted-shelled eggs. Examples of commercial layers: BV 300 (White), BV 380 (Brown), Hyline W-36, Bovans White, *etc.*

Commercial broilers are obtained by involving the White or Red Cornish, White Rock, and New Hampshire breeds. Here the male line involves Cornish strains or a synthetic population containing a variable amount of Cornish, Rock, and Hampshire blood, and a closed flock of Rock and Hampshire strains or their strain crosses are used as the female line. Examples of commercial broilers: Vencob, Cobb, Hubbard, *etc.*

68. Culling in poultry is generally based on

Answer: Performance of the bird, moulting pattern, outward appearance, pigmentation, presence of any vices *etc.*

69. Cannibalism in poultry can be taken care of by

Answer: Beak trimming, proper salt in diet, proper nutrition including minerals and amino acids, proper poultry house temperature, optimum lighting and colour of light (red/blue light), optimum feeding, an adequate amount of nest boxes, proper density of birds, culling or segregating the birds that have already developed the vice, *etc.*

70. What do you mean by FCR in broilers?

Answer: The feed conversion ratio (FCR) is obtained by dividing the amount of feed consumed by the amount of live broiler bird weight produced, *i.e.*, FCR = Total amount of feed consumed/total body weight gain. An FCR of 1.5–1.7 can be achieved with advanced genetic makeup and feed quality at 5–6 weeks of age.

71. How can you calculate FCR in layer birds?

Answer: Feed conversion ratio (FCR) is obtained by taking into consideration the feed intake, egg weight, and egg production, *i.e.*, FCR (per kg egg mass) = kg of feed consumed/kg of egg produced. FCR in layers can also be calculated by feed intake and egg production, generally calculated for a dozen eggs, *i.e.*, FCR (per dozen eggs) = Kg of feed consumed x 12/Total eggs produced. An FCR value of 1.5 or less is considered a good value.

72. Hen Day production

Answer: HDP (per cent) (for one day) = Number of eggs produced on the day/Number of birds on the day x 100

73. What do you mean by a bankable poultry project?

Answer: A bankable project involves a solid financial, economic, and technical plan, and its risk-return profile meets investors criteria and secures financing to implement the project. A bankable poultry project should be technically feasible and economically viable and includes all the assumptions as per standard market value, expenditure (recurring and nonrecurring), sale and profit and should always be vetted or signed by an appropriate authority or veterinary doctor.

A bankable poultry project involves a solid financial, economic and technical plan and its risk-return profile meets investors criteria and secure financing to implement the project. A bankable poultry project should always be vetted or signed by an appropriate authority or veterinary doctor.

74. The majority of production costs in poultry are due to

Answer: Feed cost (70-80 per cent of total cost involved)

75. Give the names of the two most important poultry feed ingredients.

Answer: Maize as an energy source and soyabeans as a protein source.

76. Which amino acid is most important for egg laying?

Answer: Methionine

77. Calcium requirement in laying hens

Answer: 3 per cent and above in the diet

78. Restricted feeding

Answer: Adopted during the growth period of layers or breeders.

79. How much feed is required for one egg production during the laying period in layer chicken?

Answer: 110-120 g/egg

80. Vitamin deficiency in chicken

Answer:

Vitamin	*Deficiency Disease*
A	Nutritional Roup
E	Crazy chick diseaseMuscular Dystrophy
K	Bleeding disease
Pantothenic acid	Chick Dermatitis
B2	Curled toe paralysis
B1	Polyneuritis/Star grazing
D	Rickets

81. Poultry hatchery

Answer: A poultry hatchery is a facility where eggs are hatched under artificial conditions in order to produce commercial day-old chicks, ducklings, or other poultry birds.

82. For how many days are chicken eggs kept in the setter and hatcher?

Answer: First 18 days in setter and last 3 days in hatcher.

83. The most common reasons for failure to hatch poultry eggs

Answer: 1. Egg storage 2. Breeder nutrition 3. Incubation faults 4. True infertility (flock age) 5. Bacterial and mold contamination 6. Genetics 7. Egg faults and shell damage 8. Disease

84. What do you mean by "post mortem"? What precautions should be taken during poultry PM to prevent any health hazards?

Answer: Postmortem, also known as autopsy, refers to an examination, investigation, or process that takes place after death. A postmortem examination of a body is often needed to determine the time and cause of death.

While performing PM on poultry, precautions should be taken to minimise exposure and ensure that personal protective equipment (PPE) is worn. Special precautions should be taken against any suspected zoonotic disease. The carcass should be handled, sampled, dressed, and disposed of in accordance with standard protocols.

85. What steps should be taken to prevent heat stress in poultry?

Answer: Poultry birds are very prone to heat stress due to their normally high body temperature (105-107°F), absence of sweat glands, feathered bodies, fatty natures, *etc.*, and steps should be taken to prevent heat stress. Proper ventilation, continuous fresh water supply, appropriate lighting, roof sprinklers or foggers in low humid areas, adequate bird density, nutritional measures like proper amino acids, bicarbonates, good quality protein, feeding birds in the cooler part of the day, providing electrolytes, vitamin C, selenium, *etc.*

86. What should be the orientation of poultry houses?

Answer: In a tropical hot humid area, the long axis of the poultry house should be in East-West direction whereas in cold/temperate weathered areas the long axis of the house should be in North-South directions. In India majority of the year in most of the areas we find hot humid weather conditions, so the long axis of poultry houses should have East-West direction to prevent direct sunlight on birds in these areas.

87. What do you mean by "integrated duck farming"?

Answer: Integrated duck farming actually refers to combining duck farming with different types of animal or plant cultures or both, such that waste produced in one operation breaks the cycle of waste by recycling it into valuable material in another. Integrated duck farming may lead to improved economic status and efficient farming. Duck integrated farming may include namely duck–rice–fish farming, duck–fish farming, duck–rice farming, and duck–rice–fish–azolla farming. In duck-cum-fish farming, duck droppings serve as feed for fish, and some fish in turn become food for ducks, whereas in duck-cum-rice farming, ducks are raised in rice fields and feed on insects, fish, and other creatures, as well as continuously stir the water in the field, preventing weed growth and improving rice growth and yield.

88. What do you mean by integration in the chicken broiler industry?

Answer: Integration was implemented in India's broiler industry few years back; however, it is not yet fully integrated. The production of broilers is integrated from the main breeder farm to the commercial grower farms. In order to obtain a fair price for broilers and to avoid middlemen's exploitation, our integrators might pursue forward integration with processing factories, marketing channels, rendering plants, *etc.*

89. All-in, all-out system

Answer: The farm will only have one batch of broilers from the same hatch under the all-in, all-out system. The number of chicks needed to fill the farm's capacity will be bought, raised, and sold as a single lot. With reduced horizontal disease transmission, subclinical illnesses, and poorer development rates, this approach is more hygienic and improves feed efficiency. This approach requires more fixed and working capital per bird, making it unsuitable for large-scale farming.

90. Environmentally controlled housing for poultry

Answer: The internal environment in the house is kept as close as feasible to the physiological requirements of the birds for peak performance.

91. Biosecurity in poultry farms

Answer: "A set of management practices which reduce the potential for the introduction and spread of disease-causing organisms on to and between sites". Poultry farms may follow proper biosecurity measures including

a) Locational biosecurity: This includes the proper location of farms away from other farms, human locality *etc.*

b) Structural biosecurity: Proper construction of sheds, a minimum distance between sheds (150 ft between brooder and grower house, *etc.*), disposal pit *etc.*

c) Operational biosecurity: Day to day operations including the procurement of chicks, proper testing of feed ingredients, minimizing handling *etc.*

d) Continuous Biosecurity: Limiting people's movements, using disinfectants, avoiding visitors, *etc.*

92. Advantages of the Californian cage system

Answer: Californian cages offer a larger feeding area. As a result, all four birds can eat at once, as opposed to traditional cages where only three birds can eat while the fourth waits in the back. Because of the shorter rolling distance, there are fewer cracked eggs and Californian cages have better ventilation than traditional cages.

93. Advantages of the deep litter system of poultry rearing in regards to nutrition of birds

Answer: Vitamin B2 and Vitamin B12 are made available to the birds from litter by bacterial action on the litter.

94. Built up litter

Answer: Deep litter or built-up litter is the accumulation and decomposition of litter material and excreta till it reaches a depth of 8" to 12", after an initial start of 3" to 5" depth.

95. How are day old chicks fed just after their arrival on the farm?

Answer: First of all, provide fresh drinking water or water mixed with electrolytes, glucose, and vitamins in waterers. Sugar or jaggery may be added to the water to provide instant energy, often 8 per cent sugar solution containing 1 per cent sodium chloride are given to chicks. Then spread ground maize or rava/suji, or fine mash or crumble feed on the old newspaper for 1 or 2 days. Afterwards, they will learn to consume feed from the feeder.

96. Lighting schedule to be followed for layer birds

Answer: From week 21 *i.e.*, at the sexual maturity of birds, start with 14 hours of light. A gradual rise of 15 minutes per week to a maximum of 16 hours, which is maintained up to 42 weeks. At 43 weeks, increase to 17 hours of light and then maintain the same. Light after 17 hours is not cost-effective in poultry houses. The light intensity at the level of the bird's eyes is crucial for promoting egg formation (0.9 to 1.2 fc). For a 3.5 m^2 floor space, a 40-watt bulb with a reflector held 2.2m above the ground delivers the appropriate intensity.

97. Beak trimming

Answer: Removal of 1/3 to ½ of the beak in poultry prevents feather pecking, feed wastage, and cannibalism. Done with the help of a hot blade beak trimmer, infrared beak trimmer, *etc.*

98. Which egg is more nutritious- a desi or backyard chicken egg or a commercial chicken egg?

Answer: Literally, there is not much difference between the nutrition value of a desi/backyard poultry egg and a commercial poultry egg of same weight. All eggs are nutritionally similar and contains the same number of vitamins, minerals, proteins and calories. In desi egg yolk, xanthophylls pigment (which converts to vitamin A) is higher due to varied feed intake, so it seems deep yellow. Whereas in a commercial egg, vitamin A is directly present, obtained from balanced feed, and the yolk seems light yellow.

99. What is the ICMR recommendation for poultry meat and egg consumption?

Answer: ICMR recommendation is 180 eggs per person per year and 10.8 kg poultry meat per person per year.

100. What are the requirements during the incubation of an egg in an incubator?

Answer:

a) Temperature: Setter temperature 99.50–99.75°F and hatcher temperature (last 3 days) 98.50°F,

b) Relative Humidity: First 18 days between 55-60 per cent and last 3 days 65-75 per cent,

c) Ventilation: Proper ventilation is to be maintained, and oxygen should be at a level of 21 per cent and carbon dioxide tolerance at 0.3 per cent.

d) Position of eggs: Eggs should be placed with the broad end up in the setter.

e) Turning of eggs: Eggs should be turned at least eight times a day in a setter, but modern-day incubators turn eggs every hour at a 45-degree angle. Turning is not required in the hatcher.

101. Name the best layer and best meat-type chicken breeds.

Answer: Leghorn is the best egg producer, and Cornish is the best meat breed.

102. What are the features of the RIR breed?

Answer: The most common colour is red buff, characterized by a long body, broad and deep breast carried well forward, a flat back, red eyes, and red ear lobes. Legs and feet are deep yellow but may show brown colour. It's a dual-purpose breed with an annual egg production of 180–200 eggs. Often, this breed is distributed in different government schemes in West Bengal, where it is popularly known as Lal Murgi (red chicken).

103. What are the characteristics of indigenous poultry breeds?

Answer: Hardiness, higher resistance to common diseases, heat tolerance (frizzled feathers, naked neck, dwarf) fibriomelanosis, good scavengers, broodiness, and the ability to hatch their own chicks, can protect themselves from predators, low input cost and relatively less production in comparison to commercial breeds available.

104. Organ where feed is initially stored for moistening and little enzymatic activity in poultry birds.

Answer: Crop

PART E: PIG

1. One of the most intelligent domestic animals.

Answer: Pig

2. A female pig that has produced a young one

Answer: Sow

3. A castrated male pig

Answer: Barrow

4. Act of giving birth to piglets

Answer: Farrowing

5. Uncastrated male pig of more than six months of age

Answer: Boar

6. Average gestation period in pigs

Answer: 3 months 3 week 3 days or 114 days

7. Berkshire breed of pig

Answer: Black in colour with 6 white points.

8. Name the domestic animal that stores fat at the highest rate per unit of live weight.

Answer: Pig

9. Importance of guard rails in farrowing crates.

Answer: Guard rails are placed 25 cm above the floor and wall to prevent crushing of piglets by the mother sow's body during movement.

10. It is good to clip of all eight needle teeth in piglets.

Answer: As a good management practice, teat injuries in recently farrowed sow can be prevented by clipping all needle teeth.

11. Castration in pigs is generally done by which method?

Answer: Surgical open method

12. Piglets are highly susceptible to which disease?

Answer: Anaemia

13. Name the highly productive native pig breed of West Bengal.

Answer: Ghoongroo

14. What measures should be taken to prevent piglet anaemia?

Answer: Injecting piglets with iron dextran injection at 100–150 mg/pig (I/M) in the neck or ham area is one of the best measures. Swabbing/painting of the sow's udder with ferrous sulfate solution and sugar from birth until the piglet starts taking creep feed, sprinkling soil soaked with ferrous sulfate (500g) and copper sulfate (75g) in 3 liters of water in the farrowing pen, allowing piglets access to a clean area of soil, or providing 4 ml of 1.8 per cent ferrous sulfate solution to the piglets every day, are all recommended.

15. Which livestock have one of the highest dressing percentages?

Answer: Pig (65-80 per cent)

16. Swine fever vaccine

Answer: First at 2 months age and needs regular booster

17. Normally weaning in pigs is done at what age?

Answer: 56 days

18. How many teats are there in sow?

Answer: 6-7 pairs

19. What are the advantages of pig farming?

Answer: Pigs have a short generation interval, are prolific (large litter size, *i.e.*, 8–10 or more), have a good FCR (3.5–4), have a great ability to convert feed into high value animal fat, and require minimum management and care.

20. On a farm, what identification methods are generally used for piglets?

Answer: Ear notching or ear tagging

21. Is artificial insemination practiced in pigs?

Answer: Yes, this is mostly done using fresh, diluted semen.

22. How can you prevent cannibalism in pigs?

Answer: Pigs should be provided adequate space and a balanced diet. Avoid stress in pigs by causing the minimum disturbance; special care should be given to recently farrowed sows, and there should be provisions for guard rails in the farrowing pen.

23. Are pigs susceptible to heat stress?

Answer: Pigs have a less number of sweat glands; they generally have high body fat covering along with a high body weight, and their thermoregulatory mechanism is not well developed, which leads to pigs being highly susceptible to heat stress.

24. Pigs are

Answer: Omnivores, monogastric and even-toed ungulates.

25. When should a sow bred after farrowing?

Answer: Most preferably in the first estrus, 4-9 days after weaning.

26. Wallowing is behaviour is common in which domestic animal other than buffalo

Answer: Pig

27. Chromosome number of domestic pigs (2N)

Answer: 38

28. Pigs are hard on pasture

Answer: As they have a rooting habit.

29. Pig production systems

Answer: The pig production system in India is scavenging (free range), semi-intensive and intensive system.

30. Pig housing

Answer: Sty (sties, plural)

31. In which group of pigs restricted feeding is not practiced?

Answer: In pigs weighing less than 45 kg.

32. Why are piglets prone to piglet anaemia?

Answer: Piglets require a minimum of 5-10 mg of iron per day, but they are born with a little reserve of iron *i.e.*, 50 mg in the liver and sow milk contains a negligible quantity of iron. So, due to the deficiency of iron, piglet anaemia is common.

33. What do you mean by "creep feeding"?

Answer: Creep feeding is the practice of self-feeding concentrate to piglets in a separate area away from the dam.

34. How much semen is ejaculated by a boar?

Answer: 100-500 ml of semen containing 30×10^9 to 150×10^9 sperm over a period of between 1-15 minutes.

35. What is Flushing?

Answer: Around 10 days before mating sows (@20g feed/kg body weight) and gilts (@5-30g feed/kg body weight) are given a good grower ration known as flushing for higher ovulation, regularity in heat, better fertilisation and subsequent proper implantation of zygote.

36. Parakeratosis in pigs occurs due to -

Answer: Deficiency of Zinc

37. Boar odour in meat is found due to -

Answer: Due to skatole and androsterone

38. What is the most important emerging disease in swine in India presently?

Answer: African Swine Fever is highly contagious and haemorrhagic viral emerging disease in India with high lethality caused by Asfivirus.

39. Labour to pig ratio in a pig farm

Answer: 1:40 with 2-3 extra laborers who may be engaged in farm activities.

40. Species of pig

Answer: Porcine

PART F: LABORATORY ANIMALS

1. What do you mean by laboratory animals?

Answer: Animals used in laboratories for scientific testing, experimentation, and research are known as laboratory animals. These animals can include mice, rats, rabbits, guinea pigs, hamsters, dogs, cats, and non-human primates, among others. They are frequently developed especially for study and put through a variety of experimental processes like drug testing, genetic engineering, and behavioral research. Ethics rules govern the use of laboratory animals to make sure that it is appropriate and that the animals are treated decently.

2. The most popular model mammalian laboratory animal

Answer: Mice

3. The most frequently used strain of laboratory mice

Answer: The C57BL/6 strain of laboratory mice is the most widely used strain in scientific research. This strain serves as a useful model organism for research into numerous diseases, genetics, behaviour, and medication development because of its well-known consistent and reproducible behaviour and genetics.

4. Adult laboratory mice weigh

Answer: 30 grams with around 2 ml of blood volume.

5. How is a small laboratory animal like mouse or rat identified?

Answer: The identification of small laboratory animals like mice and rats can be done in a number of ways. The most popular technique involves inserting tiny pieces of plastic or metal called ear tags or ear punches into the animal's ears. These punches or tags can be individually coloured or numbered to allow each animal to be identified. Other methods of identification include tattoos or dyes applied to the animal's skin or fur, or microchip implantation under the animal's skin.

6. How do you handle laboratory animal like mice and rats?

Answer: To protect the safety of the animals and the handlers, sufficient training and care must be taken when handling rats and mice in laboratories. Following are some general recommendations for treating lab rats and mice:

a) Using proper rubber gloves, and if needed use proper personal protective equipment (PPE).
b) The animals should be approached calmly and gently.
c) The animal should be picked up by handling the base of the tail.
d) The animal should never be squeezed.
e) Use proper handling techniques based on the experimental need and type of animal.
f) The health and behavior of animals should always be assessed before handling.

7. Can Guinea pigs synthesize vitamin C?

Answer: No

8. Individually Ventilated Cage (IVC)

Answer: It is a form of caging system used for research animals, mainly rodents like mice and rats. By providing a specific air supply and exhaust system for each cage, IVC systems offer a controlled and isolated environment for each animal. Each cage in IVC systems is typically constructed of transparent polycarbonate, allowing for visual animal monitoring. To keep the air supply clean and free of pathogens, dust, and other contaminants, the cages have a filter top. Also, each cage has its own ventilation system, which aids in keeping the animals healthy and halting the transmission of disease.

9. Nutrition of laboratory animals

Answer: For the health and welfare of laboratory animals, proper feeding is crucial. Laboratory animals are frequently fed specially made diets that are devoid of toxins and other dangerous chemicals, but still suit their nutritional needs. Species, strain, age, sex, and reproductive state of laboratory animals can all affect their individual dietary needs. In general, laboratory animals need a balanced diet that includes protein, fat, carbs, vitamins, minerals, and water. There are numerous commercial diet formulations for lab animals, such as pelleted or powdered diets. The diet of laboratory animals can also contain fresh fruits and vegetables, especially for herbivorous species like rabbits and guinea pigs. These items can improve and diversify the animal's diet by adding extra vitamins, minerals, and fiber. It is crucial for researchers to monitor the body weight, physical condition, and overall health of laboratory animals to ensure that they are receiving appropriate nutrition.

10. Gestation period of common laboratory animals

Answer: Rat gestation period is 21 days, Mice gestation period is 21 days, Guinea pig gestation period is 68 days, and Rabbit gestation period is 30 days.

11. SPF

Answer: SPF stands for Specific Pathogen Free. It alludes to lab animals free of particular pathogens, which are characterized as bacteria that might cause disease. The pathogen-free state of SPF animals is maintained by raising them in a controlled setting, such as a barrier facility, to avoid exposure to pathogens. However, it is important to note that SPF status does not guarantee that the animals are free from all potential pathogens.

SPF eggs are often used for vaccine development. SPF eggs are used to produce certain types of viral vaccines, such as influenza vaccines and some types of veterinary vaccines.

12. Gnotobiotic animals

Answer: Animals in which certain known strains of bacteria or other microorganisms are present are known as gnotobiotic animals. The animal is often reared and kept in a sterile isolator, which is a specialized setting that forbids exposure to any microbes, in order to produce a gnotobiotic animal. The animals are given sterile food and drink, and the isolator is fitted with HEPA filters to remove any potential contaminants from the air. In order to research how these microorganisms, affect the host, gnotobiotic animals may also be colonised with a specific set of microorganisms, such as particular bacteria or viruses.

13. What measures would you employ to guarantee the welfare of laboratory animals?

Answer: The utmost focus should be on ensuring the welfare of experimental animals. Measures like providing them with the right food and housing, reducing their stress and discomfort during experiments, and giving them the right anesthetic and painkillers when needed. One should adhere to specific protocols and rules for the use and care of animals that have been established by regulating bodies and institutions. CPCSEA guideline for Good Laboratory Practices should be followed. The concept of 4R^s may be followed.

14. What do you mean by 3R^s or 4R^s?

Answer: The concept of 3R refers to the ethical principles of replacement, reduction and refinement as introduced by the British scientists William Russell and Rex Burch in 1959 as a guide for researchers to minimize animal use and suffering in experiments and recycle the use of animals in scientific research. The recently introduced 4th R stands for rehabilitation.

15. Where from should one take permission for experimenting on laboratory animals in India?

Answer: In India, permission to experiment on laboratory animals is regulated by the Committee for the Purpose of Control and Supervision of Experiments on Animals (CPCSEA). The Prevention of Cruelty to Animals Act, 1960 allowed for the establishment of the CPCSEA, an official organization under the Ministry of Environment, Forest and Climate Change (MoEFCC), in 1964. In addition to obtaining permission from CPCSEA, the researcher must also obtain approval from their institutional animal ethics committee (IAEC). The proposed experiment must adhere to ethical standards, and the IAEC is in charge of making sure the animals will be treated humanely. India strictly enforces regulations on animal experimentation, and the use of animals in research is only authorized when it is judged necessary and when no other options are available.

16. What do you mean by animal welfare?

Answer: According to the Terrestrial Code, animal welfare means 'the physical and mental state of an animal in relation to the conditions in which it lives and dies.'

In other words, animal welfare refers to the physical and psychological well-being of animals, particularly those kept by humans for various purposes such as companionship, food, research, entertainment, or work. It involves ensuring that animals are not subjected to unnecessary harm, suffering, or distress, and that their basic needs for food, water, shelter, and veterinary care are met. Animal welfare is a significant ethical and scientific issue, and it is frequently governed by rules, regulations, and laws that are designed to safeguard animals from cruelty and ensure their welfare.

17. The "five freedoms"

Answer: "Five Freedoms" are a set of animal welfare standards that were first developed by the UK Farm Animal Welfare Council in 1965.

a) Freedom from hunger, malnutrition and thirst.
b) Freedom from fear and distress.
c) Freedom from discomfort.
d) Freedom from pain, injury, or disease.
e) Freedom to express normal behavior.

18. What is the difference between animal rights and animal welfare?

Answer: Animal welfare is concerned with promoting the well-being of animals and reducing their suffering, while still allowing for their use by humans. On the other side, animal rights contest the ethics of utilizing animals for human advantage and aim to provide animals fundamental rights and freedoms.

PART G: EQUINE AND CAMEL

1. What are Equine Species?

Answer: Equine includes horse, donkey, zebra and mule that are used for work and as pack animals.

2. State the main features of Equines.

Answer: Equines are monogastric and hindgut fermenters.

3. Breeds of indigenous horses/ponies

Answer: Marwari, Kathiawar, Manipuri, Bhutia, Spiti and Zanskari.

4. Mules

Answer: Hybrid born due to the mating of Jack (donkey) and Mare (horse).

5. Horses are kept in (housing)

Answer: Stable

6. Optimum breeding time in horses

Answer: 2-3 days after the appearance of heat

7. Gestation period of horse

Answer: 340 days

8. **Important diseases of horses**

   Answer: Glanders, Strangles, Tetanus, Pink eye, African Horse Sickness *etc.* Monday morning sickness, colic and lameness are important health issues for horses.

9. **Types of gaits in horses**

   Answer: Walk, trot, canter, pace, gallop or run.

10. **Why do horses sleep in standing position?**

    Answer: Horses can lock their leg joints ('check' ligament is present in their hip joint), allowing them to stand up straight without using any muscles to maintain balance. For their survival in the wild, horses' ability to rest and nod off while not entirely lying down is a benefit. Standing while they sleep enables horses to remain awake and prepared to respond rapidly to any perceived threat or danger. Sleeping while standing is a normal activity for horses, even though they can and often do lie down to sleep, especially when they feel safe and confident in their surroundings.

11. **Why horses can't vomit?**

    Answer: Horses are unable to vomit because of the cardias or "Swiss tie" valve at the stomach's opening, whose muscles are so powerful that they prevent food from returning to the mouth.

12. **Colt**

    Answer: Young male horse under three years of age

13. **Gelding**

    Answer: A *gelding* is a castrated male *horse* or other *equine*, such as a pony, donkey or a mule.

14. **Foal**

    Answer: A foal is an equine up to one year old

15. **Foaling**

    Answer: Act of parturition in horse.

16. **Filly**

    Answer: A young female horse before foaling is called filly.

17. **Mare**

    Answer: Adult female horses are called mare.

18. **Stallion**

    Answer: A stallion is a mature male horse that has not been gelded and used for breeding.

19. Ponies

Answer: Smaller breed of horse used for riding and driving. Height at withers is 14.2 hands and adult weight of around 136-400 kg.

20. Breeding farm of horses is known as –

Answer: Stud farm

21. Colic in horse

Answer: Colic in horses refers to abdominal pain, which may have a variety of causes such as digestive disorder, impaction and blockage in the intestinal tract. Proper treatment and management should be done at the earliest.

22. Camelidae species

Answer: Along with Camels includes Lama, Alpaca, Vicuna and Guanaco.

23. Double humped camels are found in which area of India?

Answer: Ladakh area

24. Two species of camel

Answer: Single humped *Camelus dromedarius* and double humped *Camelus bacterianus.*

25. Camels are classified into two classes

Answer: Baggage and riding type.

26. Ship of the desert

Answer: Camel

27. Camel breeding

Answer: Seasonal breeder and have induced ovulation.

28. What is Rut?

Answer: Also known as musth, is the occurrence of sexual heat in male camels.

29. Gestation period of the camel

Answer: 390 days

30. Camel milk

Answer: Camel milk has a higher vitamin C content, a longer shelf life, more salt, and contains insulin-like proteins.

31. Camel

Answer: Pseudo ruminant as omasum is absent.

Chapter 5

Livestock Diseases

PART A – LIVESTOCK DISEASES AT A GLANCE

BACTERIAL DISEASES

Disease	*Causative Agent*	*Susceptible Host*	*Clinical Signs*	*Lesions*	*Treatment*
Anthrax	*Bacillus anthracis*	Cattle, Buffalo Sheep, horse, pig and Human (Algerian sheeps are resistant)	1. High rise of body temp 2. Tarry coloured un-clotted blood from natural orifices. 3. Development of bloat. 4. Distressed breathing.	1. Absence of Rigor mortis. 2. Hepatomegaly. 3. Yellow gelatinous fluid in subcutaneous tissue.	Penicilin 10000unit per kg body weight twice daily.

Disease	*Causative Agent*	*Susceptible Host*	*Clinical Signs*	*Lesions*	*Treatment*
Haemo-rrhagic Septicaemia	*Pasteurella multocida* type 1	Cattle and Buffalo (young animals from 6 months to 2 years are most susceptible)	1. Subcuteneaous oedema of the head, neck, dewlap and brisket region. 2. Laboured breathing with grunting sound. 3. Profuse salivation_ Lachrymation and Nasal discharge.	1. Hepatization of lungs with deposition of serofibrinous exudates in the interlobular space. 2. Oedema and thickening of the interlobular septa. 3. Accumulation of fluid in the thoracic cavity and pericardial sac.	1. Oxytetracycline @ 5-10 mg per kg 2. Dexamethasone @1 mg/kg body wt. 3. Sulphanethazine @150 mg/kg body wt
Brucellosis	*Brucella abortus, B.melitensis, B.suis, B.ovis, B.canis.*	Cattle, Buffalo, sheep, Goat, Pig, Dog and Human	1. Abortion storm in last trimester of pregnancy in cattle. 2. Orchitis and Epididymitis in bulls. 3. Hygroma sweeling or Synovitis.	1. The affected foetal membranes are swollen and infiltrated with yellow gelatinous fluid. 2. Necrotic changes in cotyledon. 3. In the bull, necrotic orchitis associated with seminal vesicle involvement.	1. Oxytetracyclin 10mg/kg body wt 2. Streptomycin 10 mg/kg body wt

Disease	*Causative Agent*	*Susceptible Host*	*Clinical Signs*	*Lesions*	*Treatment*
Tuber-culosis	*Myco-bacterium tuberculosis, M. bovis, M. avium*	Cattle, Pig, Horse, Dog, Sheep and Goat, human	1. Gradual slow weight loss 2. Dyspnoea and painful dry cough. 3. Abdominal pain, Obstenate diarrhoea. 4. Nodules in the Udder. 5. Caseous discharge tinged with blood from uterus.	1. Tuberculous lesions consist of caseous core surrounded by necrotic tissues and the entire mass is encapsulated.	1. Isoniazid.@ 5-10 mg/kg body wt 2. Oral 300mg Rifampicin, 300 mg Isoniazide and 500 mg intramuscular Streptomycin are combinedly used
Paratuber-culosis	*Mycobacterium johnei*	Cattle, Sheep, Goat and Buffalo	1. Cardinal sign is intermittent or continuous diarrhoea. 2. Animal remains unthrifty with dry coat and without fever. 3. Faeces is dark and contains bubbles.4.Loose skin develops in the intermandibular space, dewlap and brisket region.	1. Red and oedematous Caecum and colon (Ileocecal valve). 2. Diffused thickening along with transverse and longitudinal corrugation of the intestinal wall. 3. Intestine mucosa and submucosae are infiltrated with epithelioid cells, multinucleated giant cells, eosinophil, lymphocytes, plasma cells and acid fast organisms.	1. Streptomycin sulfphate @10mg/kg body weight.

Disease	Causative Agent	Susceptible Host	Clinical Signs	Lesions	Treatment
Lepto-spirosis	*Leptospira pomona, L. canicola, L. ictero-haemorrhagiae, L. grippotyphosa*	Cattle, Horse, Sheep, Goat, pig, Dog	1. Haemoglobinurea (More common in calves) 2. Yellow clotted milk followed by agalactia (Cold mastitis) 3. Abortion and still birth in 5-9 months pregnant cows. 4. Les frequent manifes-tations are blindness and cerebral ataxia.	1. Multiple widespread haemorrhagic spots below the mucous and serous membrane. 2. Necrotic changes in kidney and liver. 3. Icterus 4. Retention of bile with infiltration of mononuclear cells in the liver.	1. Penicillin @ 10000IU/kg I/M 2. Streptomycin@ 10 mg/Kg I/M 3. Tetracycline20mg/Kg i/m 4. Corticosteroid
Listeriosis (Silage disease/ Circling Disease	*Listeroa monocytogenes*	Cattle, buffalo, sheep, Goat, Dog, Cat, Pig, horse, rabbit, Birds, Fish	1. Unilateral facial paralysis with drooling of saliva. 2. Panopthalmitis with pus in the anterior chamber of one or both eyes. 3. Circling movement on either direction (left or right) 4. Paralysis of pharynx leading to respiratory failure. 5. Abortion and retention of placenta in early pregnancy.	1. Perivascular cuffing, micro abscess, lymphocytic lepto-meningitis in the brain. 2. CSF shows cloudiness due to presence of excess globulin and leukocytes. 3. Placentitis and endometritis. 4. Yellow necrotic foci on liver, spleen, endocardium, pericardium and lungs.	1. Chlortetracycline @ 10mg/kg body wt i/m for 5-7 days 2. Penicillin @44000IU/kg body wt i/m for 7 days 3. Sulphonamide @ 100-150 mg/kg body wt i/m for 3-5 days

Disease	*Causative Agent*	*Susceptible Host*	*Clinical Signs*	*Lesions*	*Treatment*
Calf scour/ White diarrhoea	*Escherichia coli*	Calves, foals, lambs, Kids and piglets	1. Profuse loose stool with rapid peristalsis. 2. The stool is yellowish brown or greyish white with occasional streak of blood and foetid odour. 3. Tucked up abdomen, shrunken eyes, rough hair coat with rapid pulse and respiration. 4. Chronic cases show joint ill and pneumonia.	1. Hyperaemia of gastrointestinal mucosa. 2. Oedema and haemorrhages of the abomasal folds. 3. Abomasum will contain undigested curd. 4. In chronic case, suppurative changes will be in the joints.	1. Diet: Food should be withheld for 24 hrs. New born animal should be allowed to suckle the mother. 2. Fluid: Isotonic solution of ECF with Na 140, Cl 115 and HCO3 25 mcg per litter of 5 per cent glucoseSolution (50-100ml/kg iv in first 4-6 hrs followed by 140 ml/kg body wt over next 20 hrs) 3. Chemotherapy: Chloamphenical @25-50 mg/kg im

Disease	*Causative Agent*	*Susceptible Host*	*Clinical Signs*	*Lesions*	*Treatment*
Salmo-nellosis/ Paratyphoid	*Salmonella typhimurium, S. dublin, S.choleraesuis, S. abortusovis*	Cattle, Goat, sheep, pig, horse, rodents, man, fowl, dog	1. Profuse watery faeces with blood clot and mucus. 2. Frequent defaecation with abdominal pain. 3. Young animals show ataxia and recumbency additional to putty coloured faeces. 4. Enlargement of joints. 5. Pneumonia in pigs.	1. Haemorrhage and oedema in Gastric mucosa 2. Hyperaemia, necrosis and ulceration of intestinal mucosa. 3. Zebra marking in Caecum. 4. Enlargement of Liver and spleen with necrotic foci.	1. Fluid therapy 2. Broad spectrum antibiotics (Chloramphenical, Polymixin- B *etc.*)
Diamond skin disease	*Erysepalo thrixrhusio-pathiae* (*insidosa*)	Pig	1. Lateral recumbency of animal. 2. Hard faces followed by diarrhoea. 3. Conjunctivitis and vomition 4. In light skin of pig, characteristic small slightly pink to dark purple raised areas are seen. 5. In dark skin pig, palpable raised area can be seen.	1. Rhomboid urticarial lesions (Diamond skin disease) 2. In chronic case verrucose endocarditis is seen.	1. Antiserum: 5-10 ml sc per 50 lb of piglet 2. Antibiotics: Penicillin 50000IU per kg body wt. 3. Antiinflammatory drugs:Cortico-steroids like betamethasone is preferred.

Disease	*Causative Agent*	*Susceptible Host*	*Clinical Signs*	*Lesions*	*Treatment*
Actino-mycosis or Lumpy Jaw	*Actinomyces bovis*	Cattle of 4 years and above, pig, horse,Dog.	1. Hard painless circumscribed protuberance at the level of central molar teeth of the mandible or maxilla. 2. Large granulomatous mass appear on the surface of jaw followed by development of sinus tracts.	1. Pus containing granules referred as sulphur granules 2. Rarefaction and widespread destruction of mandible and maxilla. 3. Suppurative osteomyelitis of mandible.	1. Potassium iodide is used @4-8gramms daily orally. 2. NaI 15-30 gms in 250-500 ml of distilled water iv. 3. Isoniazide @ 20mg/kg body wt. I/M 4. Sinus tracts should be packed with lugol'siodine.
			3. The discharges from the tract are thick mucoid yellowish and purulent containing granules with clubbing. 4. Loss of general health due to impairment in mastication process. 5. Foul breath from mouth (Halitosis) with hypersalivation. 6. Fistulous withers and poll evil in horse.		

Disease	*Causative Agent*	*Susceptible Host*	*Clinical Signs*	*Lesions*	*Treatment*
Glanders	*Actinobacillus mallei*	Horse, Mules, Donkey	1. Catarrhal and grey nasal discharge. 2. The skin affection of lower limbs and abdomen is ascribed as Farcy. 3. Dyspnoea 4. Intermittent fever and cough.	1. Millet seed size grey or yellowish nodules on the upper respiratory tract mucosa. 2. Oedema of glottis	As per the provision of the Glander and Farcy act, positive animals must be destroyed and safely disposed.
Wooden Tongue/ Timber Tongue/ Big Head disease	*Actinobacillus lignieresi*	Cattle Buffalo and Sheep	1. Hardness of the tongue with drooling of saliva and difficulty in mastication. 2. Absces formation in posterior margin of soft palate may produce severe dyspnoea. 3. Retropharyngeal involvement produce snoring sound during respiration 4. Pus discharge from open abscess. 5. Enlargement of submandibular lymph nodes.	1. Granulomatous tissue formation which on incision expose greenish yellow firm nodules and abscesses of various size enclosing caseous or purulent masses. 2. Pus contains numerous sands like granules (Sulphur granules)	1. Surgical drainage of the abscess with application of Iodine. 2. Lugol's iodine should be injected locally. 3. NaI (10-20 per cent soln)@ 70mg/kg body wt. 4. IV 4. Streptomycin sulphate @5gm/ day im for 3-5 days.

Disease	*Causative Agent*	*Susceptible Host*	*Clinical Signs*	*Lesions*	*Treatment*
Epizootic abortion	*Campylobacter foetus*	Cattle, Buffalo, sheep, Goat, Man	1. Abortion during 4th- 7th months of pregnancy. 2. In case of late abortion Retention of the placenta is common. 3. Autolysis of aborted foetus.	1. Catarrhal inflammation of Cervix and vagina. 2. Endocarditis and mild necrosis of cotyledon. 3. Oedema of inter cotyledonary areas. 4. Focal necrotic hepatitis in lambs. 5. Gastric oedema in embryo calf.	Streptomycin @10mg per lb body wti–I/M
Strangles	*Streotococcus equi*	Equine (Young horses are mostly susceptible)	1. Animal is reluctant to eat, drink and move. 2. Serous to muco-purulent nasal discharge. 3. Cough 4. Thick yellowish creamy pus liberates from abscess.	1. Oedema and congestion of nasal mucous membrane 2. Empyema of Guttural pouch. 3. Abscess formation in pharyngeal and submaxillary lymp node. 4. Suppurative pneumonic changes in pleura.	1. Tetracycline @10mg/kg body wt. 2. Crystaline Penicillin 20000IU/Kg body wt.
Glasser's Disease	*Haemophilus suis*	Pig	1. Depression, Anorexia 2. Dyspnoea 3. Swollen and painful joint leading to lameness. 4. Arthritis may develop in chronic cases.	1. Serofibrinous or purulent exudation in pleura, pericardium, and periosteum. 2. Polyarthritis and meningoencephalitis.	1. Sulphadimidine 2. Tetracycline 3. Streptomycin.

Disease	*Causative Agent*	*Susceptible Host*	*Clinical Signs*	*Lesions*	*Treatment*
Foot Rot	*Spherophorous necrophorous*	Cattle, sheep, goat, Pig	1. Lameness 2. Decreased milk production. 3. Affected animal may kick on the ground and decline to move or tries to move on two legs. 4. In sheep, the horns may be separated.	Ulcerative changes in interdigital space.	1. Parenteral use of Sulphonamides, Penicillin, Ampicillin and tetracycline. 2. Local use of 5 per cent CuSO4, 2 per cent Formalin and Crystal violet.
Pink eye	*Moraxella bovis*	Cattle	1. Tearing from affected eye. 2. Ulceration with drooping of eye lids 3. vascularization and repair of cornea. 4. Healing and formation of scar 5. Photophobia	1. Granular growth on the conjunctiva. 2. Keratitis and conjunctivitis.	1. Opthalmic ointment containing chloramphenicol, oxytetracycline, penicillin and Streptomycin. 2. Tylosin3 Argylol 25 per cent and Protargol 10 per cent TID for 7 days. 4. Cortisone acetate 100-150 mg im.

Disease	*Causative Agent*	*Susceptible Host*	*Clinical Signs*	*Lesions*	*Treatment*
Black Quarter	*Clostridium chauvoei*	Cattle, Buffalo	1. Stiffness and lameness in the hind limb. 2. Swelling on the heavy muscles of buttock, shoulder, thigh and neck. 3. Swelling is hot and painful in early stage and become cold and painless later on. 4. The swelled part gives crepitating sound on application of pressure. 5. Laboured breathing and accelerated pulse rate	1. Yellowish exudates in the affected muscle. 2. Gas bubbles accumulate between muscle fibres. 3. Affected tissues turn black, due to haemorrhage. 4. A rancid odour emanates from the muscle.	Penicillin @ 20000-40000 IU per kg body wt, I/M
Tetanus	*Clostridium tetani*	Horse and mule	1. Prolapse of the third eyelids. 2. Saw horse appearance 3. Erection of the ears. 4. Muscle spasm. 5. Rigidity of facial muscles gives an anxious expression. 6. Spasm of masseter muscle leads to trismus or lock jaw. 7. Hypersensitivity with reflex irritability.	1. Early rigor mortis. 2. Congedtion in the spinal cord and medulla. 3. Lungs remain hyperaemia due to asphyxia. 4. Haemorrhage, loss of striation and atrophy of myofibrils. 5. Axomal sprouting, dense granules in the synaptic cleft and disintegration of Z lines.	1. Tetanus antitoxin3000-7000IU 2. Penicillin G 20000IU/kg IM 3. Chlorpromazine or Promazine 0.4- 1. 0 mg/kg i/m.

Disease	*Causative Agent*	*Susceptible Host*	*Clinical Signs*	*Lesions*	*Treatment*
Bacillary Haemo-globinuria or Red water disease	*Clostridium haemolyticum*	Cattle	1. Dry muzzle, sudden rise in body temp. 2. Suspension of rumination 3. Arched back posture. 4. Red coloured urine. 5. Mucous membrane of mouth, eye and vagina are pale and icteric. 6. Hypoxaemia is due to destruction of RBC	1. Tissues are dehydrated. 2. Quick rigor mortis. 3. Presence of infarcts in liver. 4. Pleural and peritoneal cavity are filled with blood-tinged fluid.	Penicillin 20000 IU/ kg I/M
Botulism or limber neck or Lion disease	*Clostridium botulinum*	Horse, Cattle, sheep, Goat, chick, duck, goose, turkey, pheasants, man	1. Partial or complete paralysis of muscles of locomotion. 2. Animal lies on sternal recumbency with leg folded under the body and head resting on flank 3. Excessive salivation due to paralysis of muscles of pharynx and throat. 4. Tongue is protruded out of mouth.	No characteristic macroscopic or microscopic lesion is found	Penicillin 20000IU/kg I/M

Disease	*Causative Agent*	*Susceptible Host*	*Clinical Signs*	*Lesions*	*Treatment*
Entero-toxaemia	*Clostridium perfringens Type A, B, C, D, E*	Cattle, Goat, Sheep	1. Enterotoxaemic jaundice in sheep and cattle due to type A infection give rise to intense icterus, hemoglobinemia and haemoglobinuria. 2. Lamb dysentery: Type B organism produce Alfa, Beta and epsilon toxin which cause enteritis and neural disorder. Severe dysentery with abdominal pain is seen. 3. Struc: Type C organism produces alpha and Beta toxin. Excess feeding of milk causing intestinal stasis favours the organism. Diarrhoea and abdominal pain have been seen. 4. Pulpy Kidney disease: Type D organism produce alpha toxin. Affected lamb jumps in the air fall in the ground and goes into convulsion	1. Enlargement of mesenteric lymph node and liver in type B infection. 2. Haemorrhage in Jejunum and ileum with epicardium, thymus and diaphragm in Type C Infection. 3. Diffuse reddening of abomasal mucosa subendocardial and myocardial haemorrhage beside straw coloured fluid in pericardial peritoneal and pleural. sac. in Type D infection.	Penicillin 20000 IU/kg body wt i/m
Braxy or Bradshot	*Clostridium septicum*	Lamb	Sudden death following Grinding of teeth and comma.	Necrosis of abomasum	No. satisfactory treatment is there.

Disease	*Causative Agent*	*Susceptible Host*	*Clinical Signs*	*Lesions*	*Treatment*
Joint Ill/ Navel ill/ Omphalitis/ Urachitis	*Calf: E.Coli, Proteus sp, Staphyllococcus sp., Streptococcus sp.Foal: E. coli, Proteus sp, Streptococcus sp. Lamb: Staphyllococcussp, Streptococcus sp, E. coli Piglet: Streptococcus sp, Staphyllococcussp, E. coli, Haemophilus pleuropneumoniae.*	Calf, Foal, Lamb, Piglet	1. Persistant enlargement and huge swelling of umbilicus revealing intense pain in palpation. 2. Purulent discharge from swelling. 3. Swollen, Hot and painful joints with crepitating sound on pressure.	Omphalitis, Omphalo-phlebitis and Arthritis	Streptopenicillin with Anti-inflammatory drugs should Cbe used.
Mastitis	*Staphyllococcus aureus, Streptococcus agalactiae Str. zooepidermicus, Streptococcus pyogenes, Str. faecalis, Corynebacterium pyogenes, Klebsiella sp, E.coli, Mycobacterium bovis, Mycoplasma bovis, Candida spp, IBR virus etc.*	Cattle, Buffalo, Sheep, Goat, Pig, Horse.	1. Swelling, hardness and pain in the udder as well as teats. 2. Yellow clots in the milk 3. Anorexia, Depression and high fever. 4. Tachycardia	Inflammation in mammary gland	1. Intrammamary infusion of antibiotic 2. Broad spectrum antibiotic in Parenteral route. 3. Antiseptic teat dip 4. Anti-inflammatory like corticosteroids. 5. Letting down the milk regularly.

Disease	*Causative Agent*	*Susceptible Host*	*Clinical Signs*	*Lesions*	*Treatment*
VIRAL DISEASES					
FMD	Picorna virus	All cloven-footed animal	1. Vesicles appear in the oral mucosa, inter-digital space, and udder. 2. Drooling of foamy ropy saliva with protruded tongue 3. Vesicles rupture leaving angry looking ulcers. 4. Severe pain with lameness.	1. Myocardial degeneration creates grey or yellow foci or streaks in young calves (Tigroid heart). 2. Intercellular oedema and necrosis of stratum spinosum layer of the epithelial cells.	1. Antiseptic mouth wash with Potasssium permanganate, Na2CO3 Boric acid and Glycerine. 2. Same solution can be used for foot bath 3. Broad spectrum antibiotic to control Secondary bacterial infection
PPR	Morbilivirus	Goat and Sheep	1. Profuse serous or mucopurulent nasal discharge with sneezing. 2. Watery diarrhoea with or without blood tinge. 3. Ulceration of lips and buccal cavity.	1. Necrosis and ulcerative changes in lips, gum, buccal mucosa, pharynx and oesophagus. 2. Zebra marking in rectum 3. Congestion in larynx, trachea and Bronchi	1. Fluid therapy to control dehydration 2. To stop diarrhoea, Anti-diarrhoeal powder can be used. 3. Dexamethasone can be used in case of acute respiratory problem.

Disease	*Causative Agent*	*Susceptible Host*	*Clinical Signs*	*Lesions*	*Treatment*
Bovine viral Diarrhoea	Pestivirus	Cattle	1. Polypnoaea, Tachycardia and polydipsia. 2. Mucopurulent nasal and ocular discharge with conjunctivitis. 3. Rough, Dry and crustated muzzle. 4. Foul smelling watery faeces	1. Focal areas of ballooning of the cells of stratum spinosum accompanied with nuclear keratolysis or pyknosis. 2. Coagulative necrosis in the lymph nodes 3. Destruction of Peyer's patches	1. Intravenous use of DNS/NS 2. Antibiotics should be used to restrict secondary bacterial infection.
Malignant Catarrhal fever	Bovid Herpes virus 3	Cattle and buffalo	1. Dyspnoea 2. Mucopurulent nasal and ocular discharge. 3. Photophobia and meiosis followed by blindness. 4. Offensive odour from mouth or halitosis. 5. Corneal opacity	1. Erosion and necrosis of oropharynx, buccal mucosa, hard palate and tongue. 2. Greyish circular foci on the cortex of kidney. 3. Conjuctivitis with corneal ulceration.	1. Oxytetracycline @10 mg/kg body wt can be used. 2. Aspirin 3. Vitamin A. 4. Corticosteroid

Disease	*Causative Agent*	*Susceptible Host*	*Clinical Signs*	*Lesions*	*Treatment*
Blue tongue	Orbivirus	Sheep (Young sheep under 1 yr are more susceptible)	1. Drooling of saliva and swelling of gum, lip and tongue. 2. Ulceration of Dental pad 3. Dry muzzle. 4. Bluish appearance of the tongue. 5. Coronary band is swollen and cracked. 6. Abortion in pregnant animal	1. Hyperaemia in Mouth 2. Gangrene in Tongue 3. Coronary band shows congestion. 4. Placenta in haemorrhagic	1. Localized lesions should be treated with topical antiseptic solution.
Vesicular Stomatitis	Rhabdovirus	Cattle, Horse, Pig and Donkey	1. Vesicles in the mucous membrane of mouth and tongue. 2. Ropy salivation 3. Lowering of milk yield. 4. In pig's snouts and feet also show ulcerative changes.	1. Intercellular oedema, epithelial necrosis and leukocytic infiltration in oral mucosa, feet, teat and udder.	Localized lesions should be treated with topical antiseptic solution.

Disease	*Causative Agent*	*Susceptible Host*	*Clinical Signs*	*Lesions*	*Treatment*
Ephemeral fever	Rhabdovirus	Cattle, water buffalo	1. Shivering and muscle trembling with high rise of body temperature 2. Salivation, nasal secretion and lacrimation. 3. Stiff painful muscle. 4. Fair number of cases begin to ruminate in 2nd or 3rd day.	1. Polysynovitis, tendov40ginitis, and periarthritis. 2. Congested pleura and pericardium.	Sodium salicylate, phenylbutazone, Analgin, and flunixin meglumine with antibiotics like Tetracycline are used.
Infectious Bovine Rhino-tracheitis	Bovid Herpes virus 1	Cattle	1. Acceleration of respiration and dyspnoea. 2. Muco-purulent nasal discharge. 3. Open mouth breathing 4. Sharp fall in milk yield 5. Mucopurulent discharge from vulva and vagina 6. Frequent urination 7. Ocular discharge (serous to purulent) 8. Incoordination and tremor 9. Abortion storm at 4 months of gestation	1. Necrosis on nostrils and muzzle. 2. Erosion.of nasal mucosa (Red Nose) 3. Pustules on the mucosa of vulva and vagina. 4. Cowdry type -A inclusion bodies have been observed in the epithelial cells.	Sulphonamides are used to check secondary bacterial infection.

Disease	*Causative Agent*	*Susceptible Host*	*Clinical Signs*	*Lesions*	*Treatment*
Pseudo-rabies or Aujeszky's disease	Herpes virus	Cattle, sheep, goat, pig, Dog and cat	1. Pruritis or itching in nose, eyes, ears, lower jaw, chest, udder, limbs and anal region. 2. Tremor, excitement, bellowing, rolling up and down *etc.* 3. Profuse sweating and salivation 4. Vomition, diarrhoea in pig	1. Congestion of Meanings, cerebrum and cerebellum. 2. Ganglion neuritis. 3. Perivascular cuffing and focal necrosis of grey matter.	Hyper-immune serum @5 ml through sub cut route can be given.
Cow Pox	Vaccinia Virus	Cattle, Monkey, Rabbit, Guineapig, mice and Man	1. Rumination suspended 2. Udder is swollen and hot. 3. Typical pock lesion on teat and udder. 4. In bulls, lesions appear on scrotum and inner thigh	1. Cellular proliferation and infiltration. 2. Eosinophilic inclusion bodies in epithelial cells.	Ointments containing salicylic acid, benzoic acid and povidone iodine is used

Disease	*Causative Agent*	*Susceptible Host*	*Clinical Signs*	*Lesions*	*Treatment*
Goat Pox	Capripox virus	Goat	1. Skin papules appear. 2. Papules are preceded by red macules. 3. Muco-purulent discharge from eyes and nose. 4. The mucous membrane of eyes, nose, lips, vulva and prepuce become necrotic. 5. Bronchopneumonia. 6. Gastroenteritis.	1. Haemorrhage in epidermis and oedema of subcutis. 2. Ballooning degeneration of epithelial cells, coagulative necrosis, With pyknotic nuclei and infiltration of neutrophils. 3. Inclusion bodies are found in the epidermal cells	Ointments containing salicylic acid, benzoic acid and povidone iodine is used
Swine Fever	Togavirus	Pig	1. Hyperaemia of the skin with purplish discolouration of snout, ears, abdomen, inner side of the legs. 2. Small areas of vesicular lesion followed by necrotic lesions on the edges of ears, tail, lips and vulva 3. Wobbling gait, ataxia, tremor (myocloniacongenita) 4. Occasional urine sucking 5. Purulent discharges from eyes.	1. Petechial and echymotic haemorrhages in all serous surfaces. 2. Liver is dark, congested, swollen and shaded with mottled appearance. 3. Button ulcer on the mucosa of large intestine.	Hyperimmune serum @50-150 ml per animal.

Disease	Causative Agent	Susceptible Host	Clinical Signs	Lesions	Treatment
Vesicular exanthema	Calci virus	Pig	1. Vesicles on the snout, coronary band of the feet, Dew claws, udder and teats. 2. Diarrhoea	1. Vesicles are filled with cellular material and serous fluid. 2. The epithelial cells may undergo degenerative and necrotic changes.	Hyperimmune serum
African swine fever or Wart hog Disease	Irido virus	Wild and bush hog	1. Cyanotic blotching of the skin. 2. Extreme difficulty in walking due to weakness of the hind quarters. 3. Increased Pulse and respiration. 4. Purulent naso-lachrymal secretion.	1. Sub epidermal haemorrhages resembling haematocyst with nodular pattern. 2. Intercellular oedema of the lungs. 3. Hyperaemic and hyperplastic changes in the spleen	No satisfactory treatment
Transmi-ssible Gastro-enteritis	Corona virus	Pig	1. Vomition, greenish white watery faeces. 2. Faeces may contain undigested milk and emit offensive odour. 3. Weakness, emaciation with ruffled hair.	1. Presence of curdled milk in stomach. 2. Congestion and petechiation on the mucosa of stomach and intestine. 3. Villous enterocytes are destroyed. So, there is atrophy of the villi. 4. Nephrosis of the Kidney.	1. Gut acting antibiotics or sulphonamides are used. 2. Symptomatic treatment to correct dehydration and hypoglycaemia (Intraperitoneal Glucose glycine electrolyte solution)

Disease	*Causative Agent*	*Susceptible Host*	*Clinical Signs*	*Lesions*	*Treatment*
Japanese encephalitis	Flavi virus	Cattle, Goat, Horse, Sheep, Pig (Amplifier host)	1. Prodromal stage: Fever and malaise without involvement of CNS. 2. Encephalitic stage: Coma and Convulsions 3. Late stage: Gradual recovery	1. Intense congestion and punched out necrosis of the grey matter, 2. Focal and confluent area of haemorrhage especially in the parieto-occipital cortex. 3. Meningeal and peri-vascular mononuclear infiltration.	Mannitol and steroids are to be used to manage intracranial pressure
Maedi	Lentivirus	Sheep and Goat	1. Dyspnoea 2. Increased respiratory rate. 3. Occasional cough and nasal discharge. 4. Auscultation revealed fluid in the lungs.	1. The affected lungs are abnormally large in size and weight and they will not collapse with opening of thorax. 2. Rubbery consistency of lungs with greyish or bluish colouration and pin head sized nodules. 3. Interstitial pneumonia is seen as the wall of the alveloltis are thickened.	No fruitful treatment

Disease	Causative Agent	Susceptible Host	Clinical Signs	Lesions	Treatment
Equine influenza	Myxovirus A/Equi-1 and A/Equi-2	Horse, Mule, Donkey	1. Watery to mucopurulent discharge from nostrils. 2. Dry cough, pneumonia and distressed abdominal respiration. 3. Painful cervical lymph gland. 4. Guttural pouch empyema and pharyngitis are common sequalae.	1. Bhronchiolitis. 2. Inflammatory changes in upper respiratory tract also.	Antipyretics, Antihistamines, sedative expectorant and bronchodialators are used.
Equine Infectious Anaemia	Retrovirus	Horse mule, Donkey	1. Oedema of ventral abdomen, brisket, foreleg and hindleg 2. Dyspnoea, Tachycardia and Anaemia. 3. Allotriophagia.	1. Subcutaneous oedema. 2. Submucosal and subserous haemorrhage. 3. Hepatomegaly and splenomegaly.	Whole blood transfusion followed by haematinic preparation.
Scrapie	Prion protein	Sheep, occasionally goat.	1. Hyperexcitability, nervousness, aggressiveness and Hyperaesthesia 2. Muscle tremor in head and neck. 3. Frequent and scanty urination 4. Intense itching with hind feet and biting at	1. Single or multiple vaculation in the neuron of medulla, Pons, mid brain and spinal cord. 2. Cytoplasmic degeneration in the neurons of CNS. 3. Proteinase resistant protein accumulates to form Scrapie associated	No treatment

Disease	*Causative Agent*	*Susceptible Host*	*Clinical Signs*	*Lesions*	*Treatment*
Louping ill	Flavivirus	Sheep, Goat, cattle, horse	1. Twitching of the lips and nostrils 2. Muscular tremor and rigidity of musculature of the neck and limbs. This is manifested by jerky stiff movement and bounding gait. 3. Hyperaesthesia, Torticollis posterior paresis and recumbency.	Non supportive polio encephalomyelitis.	Antisera (In febrile condition doesn't work) Sedatives
Bovine Spongiform Encephalo-pathy	Prion protein	Dairy and dairy crossbred cattle	1. Ataxia, Paresis, pruritis, incoordination in movement with restricted stride. 2. Rubbing of head and hind leg hypermetria. 3. Hard faeces and bradycardia due to increased vagal tone.	1. Discrete ovoid and spherical vacuoles in the cytoplasmic process of neurons of cortex, deep grey matter and white matter. 2. Intra cytoplasmic vacuoles in neuronal perikaryal (cytoplasm around nucleus) 3. Astrositosis throughout the CNS with gliosis and Cell death.	Amphotericin B

Disease	*Causative Agent*	*Susceptible Host*	*Clinical Signs*	*Lesions*	*Treatment*
Canine Distemper	Paramyxovirus	Dog, fox, jackal, wolves	1. Biphasic rise in temperature 2. Oculo-nasal discharge 3. Hyperkeratosis of foot pads. (Hard pad disease) 4. Vomition and abdominal pain 5. Epileptic fit and convulsion. 6. Conjunctivitis.	1. Meningo-encephalomyelitis with demyelination. 2. Eosinophilic intracytoplasmic inclusion bodies are noted in the, neurons, ependymal and meningeal cells.	Anti-canine distemper serum,1-5 ml per kg body wt, Anticonvulsants, broad spectrum antibiotics.
POULTRY DISEASES					
New Castle disease or Ranikhet disease.	Avian Paramyxovirus Type 1. It is divided into 5 groups 1. Viscserotropic velogenic 2. Neurotropic velogenic 3. Mesogenic 4. Lentogenic 5. Asymptomatic	Domestic poultry, guinea fowl, pheasant, pigeon, parrot *etc.*	1. First indication is sudden death 2. Green diarrhoea 3. Muscular tremor 4. Twisting of the neck to one side (Torticolis) 5. Paralysis of legs and wings 6. Arched position of the body (Opisthotonus) 7. Drop in egg production, soft shell eggs 8. Respiratory distress	1. Pin point haemorrhage on the apex of proventriculus. 2. Hyperplasia of Peyer's patches. 3. Conjunctivitis and keratitis. 4. Necrosis of the caecal tonsil. 5. Cloudy air sac due to air sacculitis.	1. No effective treatment is there. To prevent the disease Live Lentogeic type (LaSota, Hitchner B1, F strain *etc.*) vaccine and R2B vaccine are used.

Disease	*Causative Agent*	*Susceptible Host*	*Clinical Signs*	*Lesions*	*Treatment*
Infectious Coryza	*Avibacterium paragallinarum* (in the past known as *Haemophilus paragallinarum*)	Chicken, Guinea fowl and Pheasant	1. Facial oedema and conjunctivitis. 2. Loss of egg production (10-40 per cent) in laying birds. 3. Respiratory rales in advance cases. 4. In affected breeders, the hatchability and day-old chick quality might decline.	1. Serous to mucoid discharge in the nasal passage and sinuses.	
Infectious Laryngo-tracheitis	Herpesvirus	Older chickens (above 14wks) are more susceptible. Pheasants are also susceptible.	1. An acute respiratory disease with nasal discharge and moist rales followed by gasping. 2. Blood-stained mucus in laying birds 3. Egg production can drop 10-50 per cent but will return to normal after 3-4 weeks. 4. Mortality can vary from 50-70 per cent.	1. Haemorrhage in the trachea 2. Blood clot and false membrane formation in the respiratory tract.	

Disease	*Causative Agent*	*Susceptible Host*	*Clinical Signs*	*Lesions*	*Treatment*
Chronic Respiratory Disease	*Mycoplasma gallicepticum*	Chicken, Turkey, Duck, Peafowl	1. Young chickens (broilers or layer pullets) will show respiratory distress. 2. Increased feed conversion ratios. 3. Lack of appetite, decreased weight gain. 4. In adult birds the most common signs are sneezing general respiratory distress.	1. Cheesy yellow exudates in the trachea, lung and air sac. 2. Pericarditis and perihepatitis 3. Air-saculitis 4. Tenosynovitis and arthritis.	
Marek's Disease	Alpha herpes virus	Chicken, Turkey, Duck, Peafowl	1. The classical form: neurolymphomatosis (paralysis) with leg nerve involvement causes a bird to lie on its side with one leg stretched forward and the other backward. 2. When the gizzard nerve is involved, the birds will have a very small gizzard and intestines and will waste away.		

Disease	*Causative Agent*	*Susceptible Host*	*Clinical Signs*	*Lesions*	*Treatment*
			3. Acute Marek's disease is an epidemic in susceptible or unvaccinated flocks causing depression paralysis, mortality and lymphomatous infiltrations/tumours in multiple organs.		
Pullorum disease (Bacillary White Diarrhoea)	*Salmonella pullorum* (*egg transmitted vertical transmission- hen to chick also horizontal transmission chick to chick in hatcheries*)	Young chicks	1. It is seen in chicks below 3 weeks of age. 2. Large no. of dead in shell chicks and deaths soon after hatching. 3. Chicks crowd together in a small space, respiratory distress 4. White viscous, sticky, thick droppings that stick to the feather around the vent. 5. Young birds with lameness and swollen hock joint.	1. In chicks Peritonitis, unabsorbed yolk sac. 2. Liver swollen with haemorrhages visible on the surface 3. Small white necrotic foci are found in the liver, lungs, heart and gizzard wall. Sometimes white nodules in lungs and heart may be most prominent. 4. Caeca congested, may have semi-solid, cheesy material inside. 5. In Adult birds lesion is an abnormal ovary, ova being irregular, cystic, deformed.	1. Furazolidone 0.04 per cent 2. Co-trimaxazole 1 gm per 4 lit water for 5-7 days

Disease	*Causative Agent*	*Susceptible Host*	*Clinical Signs*	*Lesions*	*Treatment*
Fowl Typhoid	*Salmonella gallinarum*	Adult bird and young chicks (Vertical and horizontal transmission occurs)	1. Depressed, stand still, ruffled feather, closed eye 2. Respiratory distress 3. Most characteristics symptom a watery to mucoid yellow diarrhoea	1. Carcass have a jaundice appearance 2. Liver is swollen, friable and has a dark red or almost black colour. Surface has a coppery bronze shine. 3. Pericarditis with turbid yellow fluid in the pericardial sac and fibrin attached to the surface of the heart.	Furazolidone, Co-trimaxazole, Chloramphenicol, Ampicillin
Colibaci-llosis	*Escherichia coli*		1. Coliseptisaemia in young chicken or Hjarre's disease. 2. Egg peritonitis and coligranuloma in adult chickens. 3. Mushy chick disease and omphalitis lead to early chick mortality 4. Respiratory distress 5. Diarrhoea.	1. Perihepatitis 2. Peritonitis 3. Salpingitis 4. Synovitis/ Osteomyelitis/Arthritis 5. Pericarditis 6. Inflamed unabsorbed yolk with foul smell is found in the abdominal cavity 7. Yellow nodular growth in the wall of caeca.	

Disease	*Causative Agent*	*Susceptible Host*	*Clinical Signs*	*Lesions*	*Treatment*
Coccidiosis	*Eimeria tenella*: Caecal coccidiosis*Eimeria necatrix* :Intestinal coccidiosis*Eimeria brunetti, E. Maxima, E. acervullina, E. mitis, andE. praecox*		1. Bloody or mucoid droppings 2. Loss of body weight 3. Rough feathers 4. Egg production is reduced in laying birds. 5. Poor feed conversion	1. *Eimeria tenella* infection lead to enlarged caeca with clotted blood inside. 2. *Eimeria necatrix* infection leads to ballooning of middle portion of small intestine 3. White or red haemorrhagic foci on the intestine surface. 4. In *Eimeria acervuline* infection the mucosa may be covered with white plaques which tend to arrange in transverse fashion causing a ladder like appearance because of the striations.	Sulfadimethoxine and Amrolium combination @ 125 + 75 ppm in feed
Asper-gillosis	*Aspergillus fumigatus*	Young chicks are more susceptible than older bird	1. Infected chickens are depressed and thirsty. 2. Gasping and rapid breathing can be observed. 3. Mortality is variable, from 5 to 50 per cent.	1. Yellow or grey nodular lesions are found in the respiratory tract 2. Cheesy exudates are found in lungs and air-sacs.	

Disease	*Causative Agent*	*Susceptible Host*	*Clinical Signs*	*Lesions*	*Treatment*
			ENDOPARASITIC DISEASES		
Amphis-tomiasis	*Paraphistomum cervi, Cotylophoron cotylophorum, Gygantocotyle explanatum, Gastrothylax cruminifer*	Ruminants	1. Persistant foetid diarrhoea. 2. Polydipsia. 3. Submaxillary oedema and pale mucous membrane. 4. Colic in horse	Enteritis, Haemorrhage at duodenum and upper ileum	1. Oxyclozanide 18.7 mg/kg body wt orally twice in two days apart. 2. Hexachlorophene @ 7.5 mg/kg mixed with vegetable oil. 3. Niclosamide @160 mg/kg body wt
Bilharziasis or Schistoso-miasis	*Schistosoma bovis, S. indicum, S. spindale, S. nasalae, S. incognitum (S.suis), S. haematobium*	Cattle, Buffalo, Horse, Sheep, Goat, Pig, Human	1. Snoring sound during respiration. 2. Swimmer's itch or Hunters itch in Human	1. Cauliflower like growth in the nasal passage which is actually benign nasal granuloma (NASA)	1. Sodium antimonitartarate@ 1.5 mg/kg b.wt 2. Antimosan and Anthiomaline @ 1.7 mg/kg b.wt 3. Praziquantel @60 mg/kg b.wtorally.
Hepatic fascioliasis or liver fluke disease	*Fasciola hepatica, F. gigantica, F. jaksoni*	Cattle, Buffalo, Sheep, Goat	1. Acute: Sudden death in sheep with discharge of frothy blood from nostrils and anus. 2. Chronic Oedema under the mandible causes Bottle jaw condition.	1. Normochromic anaemia, eosinophilia. 2. Immature flukes in the Liver, gall bladder and bile duct	1. Triclabendazole 10-12 mg/kg b. wt. 2. Oxyclozanide 10-15 mg/kg b. wt. 3. Rafoxanide @ 7.5 mg/kg b. wt.

Disease	*Causative Agent*	*Susceptible Host*	*Clinical Signs*	*Lesions*	*Treatment*
Nodule worm disease	*Oesophastomum columbianum, O. radiatum, O. dentatum*	Sheep, Goat, Cattle and Pig	1. Persistent dark green coloured diarrhoea. 2. Humped back posture with elevation of tail. 3. Dry skin with unthrifty wool.	Pimply gut: Nodules of various sizes containing greenish or yellowish pus in the ileum and colon	1. Phenothiaxine @ 600-700 mg/kg b. wt. 2. Piperazine @125 mg/kg b. wt.3 Thiabendazole @50mg/kg b. wt.
ENDOPARASITIC DISEASES					
Husk and horse disease or Lungworm of cattle	*Dictyocaulus viviparus*	Cattle	1. Rapid shallow abdominal breathing (up to 100 per min) 2. Cough, Nasal discharge and increased heart rate. 3. Mouth breathing with head and neck stretched out. 4. Violent respiratory heave and grunt.	Bronchitis and Eosinophilia	1. Albendazole 7.5 mg/kg b. wt. 2. Fenbendazole 5 mg/b. wt 3. Febantel @ 7.5 mg/ kg b. wt 4. Ivermectin @ 0.2 mg/kg b. wt. 5. Levamisole @ 7.5 mg/kg b. wt.

Disease	*Causative Agent*	*Susceptible Host*	*Clinical Signs*	*Lesions*	*Treatment*
Tapeworm infestation	*Moniezia exapnsa, M. benedini, Thysaniezia giardi, Avitellina. spp, Stilesia hepatica, Thysaniezia actinoides, Anoplocephlaa spp.*	Ruminants and horse	1. Unthriftyness, poor coat 2. Comstipation followed by mild diarrhoea and dysentery. 3. In horse, Enlargement of belly is seen. They lie down and turn their head back with increased respiration	Generalised digestive tract leisons	1. Praziquantel @ 3.75mg/kg b.wt for Monieziaspp,@ 5 mg/kg b.wt for Thysaniezia.sp., @ 7.5 mg/kg b.wt for Avitellina sp.@15 mg/kg b.wt for Stilesiahepatica. 2. For horse, Pyrantel pamoate@38 mg/kg b.wt.
Gid or Sturdy	*Coenurus cerebralis or the intermediate stage of Taenia multiceps*	Sheep, Goat, Cattle, Horse	1. Blindness, ataxia, muscle tremors, nystagmus, excitability and collapse. 2. Headpressing and periodic epilepsy.	Cyst containing coenurus in cerebrum	Surgical drainage of the cyst.
Haemon-chosis	*Haemonchus contortus (Sheep and goat) Haemonchus placei (Cattle)*	Sheep, Goat and cattle	1. Loose bloody diarrhoea. 2. Mucous membrane of conjunctiva is pale. 3. Staggering gait with fast breathing 4. Wool quality damages. 5. In calves, severe anasarca develops.	Total mucous membrane in stomach suffers from chronic inflammation where large number of worms form a mat.	1. Albendazole, Fenbendazole, Mebendazole @ 5-10 mg/kg b.wt 2. Levamisole @ 7.5 mg/kg b.wt.

PART B – LIVESTOCK DISEASES (Q&A)

1. **Which type of vaccine and what strain is used in Brucella CP?**

   Answer: In Brucella CP Freeze Dried Live attenuated vaccine is used. Strain-19 is used here.

2. **In human which disease is produced by Brucella organism?**

   Answer: Human: Undulant Fever

3. **Milk ring test is used for diagnosis of which disease?**

   Answer: Bovine Brucellosis

4. **Name the causative organism of Japanese Encephalitis?**

   Answer: Flavi virus (Type-B) sub group of Toga viridae

5. **Who is the primary vector of Japanese Encephalitis?**

   Answer: Mosquito (Culex)

6. **Which animal is the amplifier host of Japanese Encephalitis?**

   Answer: Pig

7. **Tell the name of new emerging Zoonotic disease caused by eating fruit (Litchi, mango):**

   Answer: Nipha Virus infection.

8. **Who is the Symptomless carrier of the Nipha virus?**

   Answer: Fruit bat.

9. **Which animal is mostly affected by Nipha virus?**

   Answer: Pig and human

10. **Which is used as calfhood vaccine?**

    Answer: Brucellosis.

11. **Most common cause for heavy neonatal mortality in calves is due to**

    Answer: Calf scour.

12. **Frog like posture of cow is seen in**

    Answer: Bilateral hip dysplasia

13. **Which organism potentiates the mortality of Hog Cholera?**

    Answer: *Salmonella cholerasuis*

14. The circling movement of cattle is seen in

Answer: Babesiosis, Lactacidemia, Listeriosis

15. Protein urea is well marked in which condition of the kidney?

Answer: Interstitial nephritis

16. Cerebellar ataxia condition occurs due to

Answer: Cu deficiency

17. Laminitis is related to which metabolic disease?

Answer: Lactic acidosis

18. Pabble shaped abdomen is seen in

Answer: Vagus indigestion

19. Grey baby syndrome is associated with the over use of

Answer: Chloramphenicol

20. Atherosclerosis is due to which vitamin deficiency?

Answer: B6

21. Phoosy jaw condition is due to poisoning of which mineral?

Answer: Phosphorus

22. To avoid urea poisoning it should not be added above what percentage?

Answer: 3 per cent

23. Which species is most sensitive to snake bite?

Answer: Dog

24. Crooked calf disease is caused by

Answer: Lupinous

25. Mastitic milk pH is

Answer: Alkaline.

26. Achromotrichia is due to deficiency of

Answer: Cu

27. Which protozoa cause cutaneous eruptions in cattle?

Answer: *T. annualta*

28. Pyrexia is evident in which metabolic disorder?

Answer: Grass tetany.

29. Beastiality is punishable under which section of the IPC?

Answer: 377

30. Which is a killed Brucella vaccine?

Answer: BA 45/20

31. Bundle of faggot is

Answer: Mycobacterium

32. Chronic bacillary dysentery is caused by

Answer: *Mycobacterium jhonei*

33. Lung worm of sheep and goat

Answer: *Dictyocaulus filaria.*

34. *Paragonimus westermannii* **is also known as**

Answer: Lung fluke

35. Milker's nodule is caused by

Answer: Para pox virus

36. Corridore disease is caused by

Answer: *Thileia lawrensi*

37. Dog tapeworm is known as

Answer: *Dipylidium caninum*

38. Which is the most pathogenic fluke in poultry birds?

Answer: *Prosthogonimus ovatus*

39. Which is known as Indian liver fluke?

Answer: *Fasciola gigantica*

40. Billiaryamphistomiasis in swamp buffalo is caused by

Answer: *Gigantocotyle explanatum*

41. Gillar pittoo is caused by

Answer: Immature amphistomiasis

42. Nasal granuloma/snoring disease is caused by

Answer: *Schistosoma nasale*

43. Dhobi's itch/swimmer's itch/clam digger's itch is caused by

Answer: Non-human schistosomes and avian schistosomes

44. **Husk or hoose is caused by**

Answer: *Dictyocaulus filaria*

45. **Which is known as the lung worm of cattle?**

Answer: *Dictycaulus viviparous*

46. **Humpsore is caused by?**

Answer: *Stephanofilaria asamensis*

47. **Which is known as 'Whip worm'?**

Answer: Trichuris

48. **Anopheles acts as vector for**

Answer: *Plasmodium spp., Dirofilaria immitis, Seratia digitata*

49. **Tabanus acts as a vector for**

Answer: Anthrax, Surra and Equine infectious anemia virus

50. **Fanconis syndrome is caused by**

Answer: Old and degraded tetracycline

51. **Boiled rice like gravid segments in faeces of ruminants is due to tapeworm**

Answer: *Moneizia sp*

52. **Cucumber seed appearance of gravid segments in dog is due to tapeworm**

Answer: *Dipylidium sp*

53. **The nematode that affects young poultry birds**

Answer: *Ascaridia sp*

54. **Which lungworm has a higher prevalence in India?**

Answer: *Dictyocaulus viviparus*

55. **Drug used for the control of surra is**

Answer: Quinapyrmine sulphate, Isometamidium chloride

56. **Winter coccidiosis in cattle is associated with**

Answer: *Eimeria zuernii*

57. **The most pathogenic cooccidial species in cattle is**

Answer: *E.zuernii*

58. Which coocidial species affects goats?

Answer: *E.arlongi*

59. Pearl Eye is seen in which disease?

Answer: Marek‘s disease

60. Dwarfing and curling of chicken embryo is seen in which disease?

Answer: Infectious Bronchitis disease

61. What is the causative organism of Fowl Coryza

Answer: *Haemophyllus paragallinarum*

62. What is the causative organism of Kennel Cough?

Answer: *Bordetella bronchoseptica*

63. What is the causative organism of Fayding Puppy disease?

Answer: *E.coli*

64. What is Bence Jone‘s Protein?

Answer:A light chain of immunoglobulin

65. Turkey egg kidney and strawberry lymph nodes are lesions of which disease?

Answer: Hog Cholera or Swine Fever

66. Heart Water disease in cattle is caused by which organism?

Answer: *Ehrlichia ruminantium*

67. The milk ring test is used for the diagnosis of which disease?

Answer: Bovine Brucellosis

68. Hotis test is used to diagnose of which organism?

Answer: *Streptococcus agalactiae*

69. Button ulcers in lung and air sac are characteristics of which infection?

Answer: *Aspergillus sp.*

70. Abortion followed by retention of placenta occurs due to infection of which disease?

Answer: Listeriosis

71. Hazzare‘s disease is caused by which organism?

Answer: *E.coli*

72. Undulant Fever in man is produced by which organism?

Answer: *Brucella abortus*

73. Zebra Marking in caecum is caused by which bacterial disease?

Answer: Salmonellosis

74. Fistullous Wither occurs in which animal?

Answer: Horse (caused by both *Brucella abortus* and *Actinomyces bovis*)

75. In which disease tiger heart lesion found and in which animal?

Answer: Foot and Mouth Disease. In calf heart it is found. Calf death in FMD occurs due to myocardial degeneration.

76. What is the causative organism of FMD disease?

Answer: Picornavirus

77. Who causes the three days sickness? What is the other name of the disease?

Answer: Rhabdovirus. Other name: Ephemeral fever

78. Name the causative organism of Japanese Encephalitis?

Answer: Flavi virus (Type-B) sub group of Togaviridae

79. Who is the primary vector of Japanese Encephalitis?

Answer: Mosquito (Culex)

80. Which animal is the amplifier host of Japanese Encephalitis?

Answer: Pig

81. Who causes circling disease?

Answer: Listeria

82. Excess silage feeding causes which bacterial disease in cattle?

Answer: Listeria

83. Who causes Shipping Fever? What is the other name of shipping fever?

Answer: *Pusturella multocida*. Other name Haemarrhagic septicaemia.

84. What is Post partum haemoglobinurea? How it occurs?

Answer: Due to phosphorus deficiency just after parturition in high yielding Cattle.

85. Which agent causes Texas fever?

Answer: *Babesia bigemina*

86. Dollar spots in flank region of horses are caused by

Answer: *Trypanosoma equiperdum*

87. The chronic form of *Trypanosoma evansi* **in camel is called**

Answer: Tibersa

88. 'Turning Sickness' in cattle is associated with

Answer: *Trypanosoma theileri*

89. Gall sickness and jaundice is associated with disease caused by

Answer: *Anaplasma marginale* in cattle

90. Storms of abortion in sheep is caused by

Answer: *Toxoplasma gondii*

91. Pimply gut/Knotty gut in sheep is caused by

Answer: *Oesophagostomum columbianum*

92. Cooly's itch/water itch/ground itch is caused by

Answer: Ancylostomiasis

93. The specific lesions in the liver caused by fascioliasis are

Answer: Pipe stem liver

94. Chronic fascioliasis of cattle exhibits

Answer: Submandibular edema/bottle jaw

95. Worm nests are characteristic lesions of

Answer: Srongylosis

96. Caecal worm in poultry is

Answer: *Heterakis gallinarum*

97. Epidemic typhus is caused by

Answer: *Rickettsia prowazekii*

98. Scarlet fever is caused by

Answer: *Streptococcus pyogenes* gr A

99. Enzootic abortion in ewes is caused by

Answer: *Chlamydia abortus* and *Chlamydophila abortus*

100. Lumbar paralysis in dogs is associated with

Answer: *Hepatozoon canis*

101. Blue tongue in sheep is transmitted through

Answer: Culicoides mosquito (Semen, Blood)

102. The most and least common serotype of FMD virus in India are

Answer: O and C respectively.

103. Total no of serotypes of Apthovirus causing FMD in animals are

Answer: Seven, *i.e.* O, A, C, Asia-1, SAT-1, SAT-2, SAT-3

104. Muscle has ' Fish flesh ' appearance in which disease

Answer: Stiff lamb disease

105. FMD is highly fatal in young calves due to

Answer: Necrotizing myocarditis/tigroid heart

106. The amplifying host of FMD viral infection is

Answer: Pig

107. Panting, hyperthermia and hair overgrowth are secondary effects of

Answer: FMD

108. Vaccination failure is more common in FMD because of

Answer: Antigenic drift of viral pathogens.

109. Haemorrhagic lesions at the junction of the proventriculus and gizzard are seen in

Answer: IBD

110. Infectious bronchitis in poultry is caused by

Answer: Avian gamma coronavirus

111. False layer syndrome with permanent damage of oviduct is exhibited in

Answer: IB

112. Femoral head necrosis in poultry is due to

Answer: Molybdenum deficiency

113. The capsule of anthrax bacilli contains an agent that prevents phagocytosis

Answer: Poly –gamma – D-glutamic acid

114. Malignant carbuncles are observed in human beings in

Answer: Anthrax

115. The ideal clinical sample to be collected for conducting Ascoli's test for the diagnosis of anthrax is

Answer: Muzzle

116. By which reaction Bacillus organisms are detected in blood smear in case of anthrax

Answer: Mac Fadyean's reaction

117. How will you conduct postmortem of an anthrax suspected carcass?

Answer: The post mortem examination is not carried out in suspected cases of anthrax as spore formation takes place upon exposure to adverse condition. The spores can survive very long in the soil and may spread the disease in the population. It has zoonotic significance.

118. 'Ras-berry jam' and 'Black berry jam' appearance of the spleen are observed in

Answer: Equine Infectious Anaemia and Anthrax

119. The methylene blue staining of blood smear from a HS patient shows

Answer: Bipolar staining

120. Which is known as symptomatic anthrax?

Answer: Black Quarter

121. Which organisms cause false Black Quarter?

Answer: *Clostridium septicum* and *Clostridium novyi*

122. Lock jaw in horses with a prolapsed 3rd eyelid is caused by

Answer: *Clostridium tetany*

123. The mode of infection and death in Tetanus is due to

Answer: Wound and Asphyxia

124. The least and most susceptible species to Tetanus is

Answer: Chicken and Horse

125. What is the etiology of Limber neck infection?

Answer: *Cl. Botulinum* A

126. Diamond shaped hyperaemic skin lesion, vegetative endocarditis and valvular thrombosis are characteristic features of

Answer: Swine Erysipelas

127. Swine Erysiepelas is caused by

Answer: *Erysipelothrix rhusiopathiae*

128. Circling disease in cattle is caused by

Answer: *Listeria monocytogenes*

129. Bumble foot in poultry is caused by

Answer: *Stapylococcus aureus*

130. Staphylococcus aureus in Pig causes

Answer: Greasy pig disease

131. Blue bag condition and botriomycosis in animals are caused by

Answer: *S.aureus*

132. Recurrent mastitis and summer mastitis are caused by

Answer: *Staph aureus* and *Arcanobacterium pyogens*

133. Which is known as Equine Plague?

Answer: African Horse Sickness

134. Equine distemper is otherwise known as

Answer: Strangles

135. Which is known as Swamp Fever?

Answer: Equine Infectious anaemia

136. Wooden tongue is caused by

Answer: *Actinobacillus lignieresii*

137. *Actinomyces bovis* **in cattle causes**

Answer: Lumpy Jaw

138. Fowl typhoid and Bacillary white diarrhoea in poultry are caused by

Answer: *Salmonella gallinarum* and *Salmonella pullorum*

139. Dry gangrene and poly arthritis in the calves is caused by

Answer: *Salmonella dublin*

140. Catarrhal enteritis, an enlarged coppry bronzed bile-stained liver with haemorrhagic necrotic foci in the spleen, kidney and vertical transmission are characteristic of

Answer: Fowl typhoid.

141. Corkscrew like morphology is seen with organisms like

Answer: Leptospira

142. Glasser's disease in pigs is caused by

Answer: *Haemophilus parasuis*

143. PPR is also known as

Answer: Goat plague and Stomatitis-Pneumoenteritis

144. Zebra marking in intestine with necrosis of lymphocytes in Peyer's Patches and lymph nodes and shooting diarrhoea are characteristics of

Answer: Rinder Pest

145. Which is usually a feature of PPR but not observed in RP?

Answer: Pneumonia

146. The pathogen that causes foot rot,calf diphtheria and necrobacillosis is

Answer: *Fusobacterium necrophorum*

147. Hog Cholera (swine plague) is caused by

Answer: Pesti virus

148. Turkey egg appearance of kidney and button ulcer in colon are characteristic lesions of

Answer: Classical swine fever

149. Pseudorabies of pigs is otherwise known as

Answer: Aujeszky'sdiease, Mad itch, Infectious bulbar paralysis

150. Petechial haemmorrhage at the tip of proventricular gland are pathognomonic lesion of

Answer: Ranikhet disease

151. Newcastle disease in poultry is caused by

Answer: Paramyxovirus

152. Which clinical form of RD is highly virulent and causes mortality in chicken?

Answer: Viscerotropic vellogenic (Doyle's form)

153. The most pathogenic coestode of poultry is

Answer: *Davainia proglottina*

154. Salt and pepper appearance of small intestine of poultry with white foci is observed in

Answer: Coccidiosis

155. Lumpy skin disease of cattle is caused by

Answer: Capripox virus

156. ORF is caused by

Answer: Pox virus

157. Transmissible gastroenteritis in pigs is caused by

Answer: Corona virus

158. Q fever is caused by

Answer: *Coxiella burnetti*

159. A cow is suspected to suffer from milk fever if its serum calcium concentration is

Answer: <5 mg/dl

160. Shaggy heart/corrugosum is fibrinous pericarditis with 'bread and butter' appearance is an important clinical finding in

Answer: TRP

161. "Bread and butter" pericarditis is an example of which inflammation?

Answer: Fibrinous inflammation

162. Miler's disease/Big head disease in horses is characterized by

Answer: Osteodystrophia fibrosa, excessive bran feeding, Ca:P is 1:2, hyperparathyroidism

163. Monday morning sickness is characterized by

Answer: Equine Rhabdomylosis, Azoturia/myoglobinuria, lactic acid in muscle

164. Histamine is secreted by which cell?

Answer: Basophils

165. The cell which acts as the first line of cellular defence is

Answer: Neutrophils

166. Antibodies are produced from which cells?

Answer: Plasma cells

167. Biphasic type of Vanden Berg reaction is observed in

Answer: Toxic Jaundice

168. What is anthracosis?

Answer: Deposition of carbon particles in the lungs

169. Eosinophils are the inflammatory cells mostly seen in what type of infection?

Answer: Parasitic infections

170. When the suppurative inflammation involves the connective tissue diffusely, it is termed

Answer: Cellulites

171. Small focal suppurative area in the hair follicle or sebaceous gland is known as

Answer: Furuncle

172. The type of giant cells that are seen in tuberculosis are

Answer: Langhan's giant cell

173. What type of necrosis seen in TB?

Answer: Caseation necrosis

174. What type of inclusion body observed in canine distemper?

Answer: Cytoplasmic and intranuclear inclusions

175. Which stain is used for the demonstration of Negri bodies?

Answer: Seller's stain

176. Define metaplasia

Answer: Transformation of one type of tissue into another is called metaplasia

177. What is Degnala Disease?

Answer: Degnala disease is caused by mycotoxins produced by different species of fungi namely *Fusarium* sp. *Aspergillus* sp. *etc.*

178. How will you manage vetero legal/wild life cases? (for PM)

Answer:

a) Both the case should not be handled without any written request from competent authority.

b) PM should be done on govt. land/property, not on any private land/ property.

c) Police personnel (For vetero-legal) and wildlife personnel (for wild life) should be preset during inspection and PM of carcasses
d) All the body parts should be handed over to the accompanying personnel.
e) PM report should be sent to the higher authority.

179. How will you deal with/prepare for a disease outbreak investigation?

Answer:

a) Precautionary measures should be maintained
b) Animal movement should be restricted
c) To inspect affected/dead animals proper protective clothing should be maintained.
d) Proper sampling from affected/dead animals is necessary for further lab. diagnosis (nasal swab. buccal swab, smear, tissues, blood, ruminal/ stomach content, parasites, faeces *etc.*).
e) A report should be sent to the higher authority.

180. The most and least common serotype of FMD virus in India are

Answer: O and C, respectively

181. FMD virus is susceptible to which chemical agent?

Answer: 4 per cent Sodium carbonate solution

182. Carrier cattle may harbor FMD virus for up to 1 year in

Answer: Oesophagial-pharyngeal fluid

183. The typical FMD vesicles are found in

Answer: Tongue epithelium, udder, buccal mucus membrane and interdigital space.

184. Tigroid heart is characteristic PM lesion of

Answer: FMD

185. Death occurs from FMD mainly due to

Answer: Myocardial necrosis

186. Animals after recovery from FMD become prone to mastitis due to

Answer: Ulcer in teats

187. The post FMD sequels are

Answer: Panting and salivation, hyperthermia, hypertrichosis, mastitis

188. The sample collected for confirmatory diagnosis of FMD

Answer: Vesicular fluid

189. FMD vaccine strains available in India are

Answer: O, A, C, Asia 1

190. The recommended initial age for FMD vaccination is

Answer: 4 months

191. Ring vaccination carried out to prevent FMD in breeding farms at a radius of

Answer: 10 Km

192. For FMD sero-surveillance the serum sample is collected after ___ day of FMD vaccination

Answer: 28 days

193. PPR is caused by

Answer: Morbillivirus of the Paramyxoviridae family

194. PPR virus may be cultivated in which cells?

Answer: The kidney cells of sheep and goats

195. Which animal is mostly susceptible to PPR?

Answer: Goats are highly susceptible while sheep are less susceptible and cattle may develop sub clinical infection

196. How PPR is transmitted?

Answer: Direct contact, inhalation, ingestion of contaminated feed and water

197. Which systems are affected by PPR?

Answer: Gastro intestinal system and respiratory system

198. What happens in GI tract infection of PPR?

Answer: Diarrhoea followed by dehydration and in extreme cases death of the animal.

199. What happens in respiratory tract infection of PPR?

Answer: Pneumonia > Respiratory distress > Anoxia > Death

200. What lesions are found in oral mucosa from PPR?

Answer: Necrotic lesions are seen in lip, buccal mucosa and gums.

201. Which samples to be collected for confirmatory diagnosis of PPR?

Answer: Faeces, nasal and ocular swab.

202. Which vaccine is used against PPR and at which age?

Answer: Tissue culture vaccine. 1st vaccine to be given at 3-4 months of age.

203. Which animal is the most potential reservoir host of Rabies?

Answer: Dog is the most potential reservoir host followed by fox

204. Name the causative organism of Rabies.

Answer: Lyssavirus of the Rhabdoviridae family

205. Where the Rabies Negribodies are found?

Answer: Hyppocampus of carnivores and Purkinjee cells of herbivores.

206. What is Babes Nodule?

Answer: Proliferated glial cell cluster caused by Rabies is called Babes Nodules.

207. What is the incubation period of Rabies?

Answer: Typically, 20-60 days in 85 per cent of cases, 3 months in 14 per cent of cases and 1 year in 1 per cent of cases. Though 19 years 6 months incubation period has also been reported.

208. What are the different forms of rabies? Describe in brief.

Answer:

a) Furious form: The behavior of dog will change. Biting tendencies towards both inanimate and animate objects will emerge. There will be altered facial expression and dilated pupils. While moving from one location to another, a rabid dog may bite people or other animals. Dog tries to lick water but is unable to swallow due to paralysis of the pharyngeal and laryngeal muscles.

b) Dumb form: This is the paralytic form. The lower jaw, tongue, larynx, and throat are all paralysed. The infected dogs are unable to bite. Excessive salivation is observed because the jaw muscle is paralysed. A typical voice known as a howl is created at this stage.

209. Is the milk of rabid animal safe for human consumption?

Answer: The rabies virus is killed by heat, so boiled or pasteurized milk from a rabid animal is safe for human consumption. Unpasteurized raw milk is theoretically considered as a source of infection, but no occurrence of developing rabies has been reported so far.

210. What symptoms are observed in rabid cows?

Answer: Incoordination of behaviour, a sharp decline in milk production, paralysis of the jaw, laryngeal, and pharyngeal muscles, drooling of saliva, and teeth grinding are all symptoms. Due to the paralysis of the jaw muscle, drinking water is difficult. Vocal chord paralysis alters voice quality. The most frequent symptoms seen in field situations are bellowing and excessive salivation.

211. What post bite measures should be taken in rabies cases?

Answer: Clean the bite site several times with soap. Alkali stops the rabies virus from spreading. In cases of dog bite, suturing of any kind should be avoided because it may encourage the spread of viruses. Iodine tincture can be used for cleaning. The area around the wound should be injected with antirabies serum (RIG). It is important to follow the proper post-bite immunization routine.

212. State the prophylactic vaccination schedule of Rabies vaccine.

Answer: For animals 1ml rabies vaccine to be injected s/c at 3 months of age and it should be revaccinated annually. Incase of human prophylactic vaccination should be conducted at 0, 7 and 21 days.

213. State the post exposure rabies vaccination schedule.

Answer: For animals 1ml s/c Injection should be given on 0, 3, 7, 14 and 28 days. The same schedule is followed for human also.

214. Which animals are most susceptible for Anthrax?

Answer: Cattle and sheep followed by goat, horse and pig

215. Why is anthrax also referred to as splenic fever?

Answer: Extreme Splenomegaly is found in PM lesion of Anthrax.

216. Which disease was found first to be caused by bacteria?

Answer: Anthrax

217. Which is the causative organism of Anthrax?

Answer: *Bacillus anthracis*

218. What are the toxins found in anthrax bacilli?

Answer: Oedema toxin, protecting antigen and lethal factor (toxin)

219. Which are the main virulence factors of anthrax?

Answer: Three component protein exotoxins and poly-D-glutamic acid capsules.

220. Why anthrax can remain endemic in a particular area for a long time?

Answer: When anthrax organisms leave the body, spores are produced. These spores are climatically resistant and can survive in soil for up to ten years. The spores are consumed by healthy animals during grazing. Under favourable condition within the body the spores can germinate to vegetative form of the bacteria and produce the disease again.

221. How animals die from anthrax?

Answer: During the onset of septicaemia, the bacterium releases exotoxins, which cause tissue oedema. Animals die at this stage due to shock and severe renal failure.

222. Why blood of dead animal died from anthrax is found tarry in color?

Answer: The anthrax bacillus consumes oxygen from blood and as a result color of blood becomes tarry.

223. What are the clinical manifestation of anthrax?

Answer: Increased body temperature (from 104° to 108° F), sudden bloat and acute depression in the animal. The heart rate and breathing rate both increase, and later on, severe respiratory distress is seen. After the death of animal blood oozes from natural orifices.

224. Name an animal resistant from anthrax?

Answer: Dog

225. What sins are found in human from anthrax?

Answer: Malignant carbuncles and pneumonia.

226. What is the drug of choice of Anthrax?

Answer: Penicillin @ 10000 IU per Kg BW.

227. Which vaccine is given to control spread of anthrax and which vaccination procedure to be followed?

Answer: Anthrax spore vaccine is given @ 1ml s/c and ring vaccination process to be followed.

228. What is the causative organism of Haemorrhagic Septicaemia?

Answer: *Pasteurella multocida* type I.

229. How HS is transmitted?

Answer: Direct contact, inhalation and ingestion of droplets.

230. Which age group of cattle are more susceptible for HS?

Answer: All age group are susceptible but adult animals are more susceptible.

231. What is the incubation period of Haemorrhagic septicemia?

Answer: Normal incubation times range from a few hours to a few days; however, some animals can carry the organism for varying times without showing any symptoms.

232. How death occurs from HS?

Answer: Histamine, prostaglandin, and certain fibroblastic components are generated as a result of the destruction of bovine mononuclear leukocytes and lung macrophages by organisms. They cause fast inflammatory changes in the lungs, leading to the development of fibrinous bronchopneumonia. Animals die as a result of toxemia and hypoxia.

233. State the symptoms of HS in cattle?

Answer: Cattle and water buffalo typically experience acute or sub-acute cases. Buffalo typically exhibits more severe clinical indications and a quicker disease course, despite the fact that the disease is quite similar in both species. First indicators could include a temperature, drowsiness, and a reluctance to move. Edematous swellings are noticeable in the submandibular region, along with salivation and a profuse, serous nasal discharge. The neck and brisket also develop edoema. In addition, there have been reports of hemorrhagic gastroenteritis in calves. With the onset of the first clinical indications, the animal has respiratory distress and frothing at the mouth before collapsing and dying most commonly 6 to 48 hours from the onset of disease.

234. What is the drug of choice of HS?

Answer: Sulphadimidene Inj. @150 mg per Kg. Oxytetracycline @ 5 to 10 mg per Kg.

235. State the vaccination protocol against HS?

Answer: For preventative vaccination against HS in cows and buffaloes with the following vaccination regimen: formaldehyde-inactivated culture of Pasteurella multocida adsorbed on Aluminum hydroxide gel is available in India.

Primary vaccination: six months of age or above, followed by booster dose after one month.

Revaccination: Annually

236. What are the common synonyms of Brucellosis?

Answer: Malta fever, Mediterranean fever, Undulant fever, Bang's disease, Enzootic abortion, Contagious abortion

237. What is the causative organism of Brucellosis?

Answer: *Brucella abortus, Brucella melitensis*

238. What are the peculiar characters of Brucella organism?

Answer: They are intracellular gram-negative rod or coccobacilli. They are aerobic but require CO2 for growth.

239. Which Brucella Spp do not require CO2 for growth?

Answer: *Brucella suis* and *Brucella canis*

240. Which animals are susceptible to Brucellosis?

Answer:

- ☆ Cattle -> *B. abortus* > *B. melitensis*
- ☆ Buffalo -> *B. abortus* > *B. melitensis*
- ☆ Human -> *B. melitensis* > *B. abortus*
- ☆ Sheep and Goat -> *B. abortus* > *B. melitensis*

241. Which age group of cattle are more susceptible to Brucellosis?

Answer: Pregnant cattle > Heifer at breeding age > Female calf

242. What are the common modes of transmission of Brucellosis?

Answer: By consuming food and water that have been contaminated with aborted fetuses, an infection can spread. Conjunctiva and skin penetration, as well as inhalation, sometimes may cause the disease.

243. Does natural service transmit Brucellosis from an infected bull to a cow?

Answer: No, as the organisms are deposited in vagina, the organisms will be destroyed.

244. Does Artificial Insemination transmit Brucellosis from an infected bull to a cow?

Answer: Yes, as the infected materials are directly deposited in uterus the organisms rapidly set up there and cause rapid infection.

245. What causes pregnant cows to be more susceptible to Brucellosis?

Answer: Foetus produces erythritol, which triggers the multiplication of Brucella organism in uterus.

246. What is the cause of abortion made by Brucella spp.?

Answer: A severe case of ulcerative endometritis is produced by the high concentration of organisms in foetal fluid and membrane. Abortion occurs in the third trimester due to ulcerative endometritis.

247. How is Brucella transmitted to new born calves?

Answer: Congenital infection through uterine route and the milk of infected animals is a potential source of organism.

248. What are the public health/occupational risks associated with Brucellosis?

Answer: Brucellosis is easily spread humans to human, resulting in an acute febrile disease, often known as undulant fever, which can progress to a more chronic form and cause major problems affecting the musculoskeletal, cardiovascular, and central nervous systems. To avoid infecting humans, precautions should be taken. Brucella is assigned to Risk group III in the World Health Organization's (WHO) laboratory biosafety handbook.

249. How is Brucellosis transmitted in human?

Answer: The greatest danger to the general public in areas where the disease is endemic, is consumption of contaminated dairy products. Infection is frequently brought on by occupational exposure and is mostly acquired by the oral, respiratory, or conjunctival pathways. Handling of sick animals, aborted foetuses, or placentas poses a risk to farmers and veterinarians in their line of work.

250. How to prevent Brucellosis? What are the vaccines available?

Answer: *Brucella abortus* strain 19 vaccine: In order to prevent brucellosis in cattle, the *Brucella abortus* S19 vaccine is most usually employed. In order to protect female calves between the ages of 3 and 6 months, it is given as a single subcutaneous dose. On the other hand, some animals may abort or excrete the vaccine strain in their milk, or acquire chronic antibody titers.

Brucella abortus strain RB51 vaccine: Some nations have utilized the *B. abortus* strain RB51 vaccination since 1996 to combat brucellosis in cattle. Regarding how effectively strain RB51 protects cattle compared to S19 induced protection, there is some controversy. In other nations it is advised to immunize cattle while they are calves. (4-12 months of age).

251. What happens if accidental exposure of Brucella vaccine occurs in humans?

Answer: The animals should be vaccinated with the utmost care. Because the strains used in vaccines are live and not entirely attenuated and may infect people. In such cases, immediate medical assistance should be required. If left untreated, RB51 and S19 both can infect people and result in an excessive fever. The RB51 strain is highly resistant to rifampicin.

252. What is the herd test of Brucellosis?

Answer: Rose Bengal Plate Test (RBPT)

253. What causes Black Quarter in bovines?

Answer: Black Quarter is most commonly caused by *Clostridium chauvoei.*

254. How BQ is transmitted?

Answer: *Clostridium chauvoei* is primarily found in contaminated grassland. In difficult circumstances, the organism produces spores that are resistant to the environment. These spores can stay dormant in the soil for years before becoming infectious when swallowed by livestock during grazing and infecting their large muscles. Huge amounts of gas are produced by growing bacteria in large muscles.

255. Which animals are susceptible to Black Quarter?

Answer: Usually BQ affecting cattle, sheep and goats.

256. What symptoms or signs can be seen in BQ affected animals?

Answer: At first, a fever may appear, and the affected limb may feel warm to the touch. The damaged limb shows obvious enlargement, and the animal becomes lame on that leg.

It is noted that there is crepitation or a feeling of air beneath the skin. Once clinical symptoms start to appear, the animal may only have a short lifespan, sometimes just 12 hours.

257. How is BQ diagnosed in animals symptomatically and clinically?

Answer: Crepitating noises and edematous swelling will be present in the rear limbs. By doing a physical examination and verifying the presence of gram-positive rods on a slide created from serous fluid collected from the location, the diagnosis is made.

258. Why black patches are developed from Black Quarter?

Answer: Bacteria invade live tissue and release toxins that leads to the death of the tissues, resulting in the development of these black patches.

259. What is the drug of choice for Black Quarter?

Answer: Penicillin is the drug of choice for treatment. Treatment is only effective in the early stages and as a control measure.

260. How to prevent BQ? What are the vaccines available?

Answer: A combination vaccine containing formaldehyde-inactivated cultures of *Pasturella multocida* and *Clostridium chauvoei* adsorbed on aluminum hydroxide gel can provide effective protection against BQ and hemorrhagic septicemia when given as a preventative measure.

Primary vaccination: six months of age or older, followed by a booster dose after one month.

Revaccination: Annually

261. What is bovine Tuberculosis (TB)?

Answer: Bovine TB is a contagious, chronic bacterial disease caused by *Mycobacterium bovis.*

262. Which animals are susceptible to bovine Tuberculosis?

Answer: Bovine TB primarily affects cattle, but it can be transmitted to any warm-blooded animal, including human.

263. What are the symptoms of bovine tuberculosis

Answer: Clinical symptoms of TB are not seen in the early stages. Emaciation, lethargy, weakness, anorexia, low-grade fever, and pneumonia with a persistent, moist cough are some clinical indications that may appear in the latter stages. Additionally, lymph nodes could expand.

264. How does an animal become infected with tuberculosis?

Answer: The bacteria that causes bovine tuberculosis can be present in affected animals' saliva and is transmitted through the air through respiratory tract-derived airborne particles. The bacterium can also be transferred by ingesting raw, unpasteurized milk from infected animals or through feed or water in areas that have been contaminated with saliva and other bodily fluids (urine, manure).

265. Can *M. bovis* survive in the environment?

Answer: *M. bovis* is highly resistant. Temperature and moisture have a significant impact on survival. Away from sunlight and in wet environments like soil and manure, M. bovis can persist for several months, especially in the cold. The bacteria die when exposed to high summer temperatures, sunlight, and dry conditions.

266. Can people get infected from bovine TB?

Answer: People may have TB infection. Drinking unpasteurized milk from a herd of diseased cows is the most likely way for humans to get infected.

267. What is the significance of Acid-Fast staining in identifying *M. bovis*?

Answer: Bacterial cell walls, a waxy material, contain mycolic acid. As it is heated, the material becomes softer, allowing the stain to enter the bacterium. Alcohol or acid do not oxidize the stain. Ziehl-Neelsen staining is the name of this method of staining.

268. Is it possible for tuberculosis to be transmitted sexually?

Answer: Yes, tuberculosis can be transmitted via genital tract during coitus. Also, the disease may be transmitted from infected bulls through artificial insemination.

269. What is Tubercle and where is it found?

Answer: The tuberculous lesions consist of caseous core surrounded by necrotic tissue and the entire mass is encapsulated with tissue. Tubercle refers to these nodular TB-produced structures. Although it affects all of the thoracic organs but the liver and lung are most frequently affected.

270. What is Tuberculin?

Answer: Tuberculin, also known as purified protein derivative, is a combination of proteins that are used in the diagnosis of tuberculosis.

271. What is the drug of choice for Bovine tuberculosis?

Answer: Streptomycin, Isoniazid, Rifampin

272. What is BCG vaccine?

Answer: Bacillus-Calmette–Guerin (BCG) vaccine is a vaccine primarily used to prevent tuberculosis (TB). It is named after its inventors Albert Calmette and Camille Guerin.

273. What is Johne's disease? Name the pathogenic organism.

Answer: Johne's disease is known as Para Tuberculosis of ruminants and is characterized by severe fatal gastrointestinal disorder, progressive emaciation and diarrhea. Causative organism is *Mycobacterium paratuberculosis.*

274. Which animals are susceptible to Para Tuberculosis?

Answer: Cattle and buffalo are most susceptible but sheep and goats are also susceptible.

275. Which organ is mostly affected by Para Tuberculosis and what are the common signs and symptoms?

Answer: GI system is affected. The most cardinal sign is intermittent or continuous diarrhoea.

276. What are the common causative organisms of Leptospirosis?

Answer: *Leptospira Pomona, L. canicola, L. icterohaemorrhagia etc.*

277. What is the mode of transmission of Leptospirosis?

Answer: Direct contact with urine of infected animals or ingestion of urine contaminated feed and water.

278. What is "Cold Mastitis"?

Answer: With yellow clotted milk agalactia, elevated temperatures are seen in milking cows with Leptospirosis infection. This condition is called as Cold Mastitis.

279. Is abortion related with Leptospirosis? When it occurs?

Answer: Yes, abortion and still birth are seen in pregnant animals affected by Leptospirosis in the 5th to 9th month of pregnancy.

280. What is the treatment of Leptospirosis?

Answer: Penicillin, Streptomycin or Tetracycline for 5 to 7 days.

281. What is Silage disease?

Answer: Listeriosis is known as Silage disease. Also known as Circling disease or Meningo-encephalitis.

282. How is Listeriosis spread and who are the susceptible host?

Answer: Potential infection sources include contaminated feed and soil. Additionally, silage has been identified as a significant disease spreader. The susceptible hosts are cattle, buffalo, sheep, goats, horses, and pigs.

283. What are the predisposing factors of Listeriosis?

Answer: Nutritional deficiency, heavy silage feeding, abrupt change in weather, long period of flood.

284. What are the most common symptoms of Listeriosis?

Answer: Animals with encephalitis rub their heads against hard surfaces, exhibit unilateral facial paralysis, salivation, conjunctivitis, nasal discharge, and eventually exhibit circling movements.

Abortion: Abortion is also seen and after an abortion, it's common for the fetus to be retained. Abortion occurs in early pregnancy.

Septicaemia: It is common in new born calves.

285. What is the causative organism of Wooden Tongue?

Answer: *Actinobacillus lignieresi*

286. Which are the susceptible host of *Actinobacillus lignieresi?*

Answer: Cattle, buffalo and sheep.

287. What is the treatment of Wooden tongue?

Answer: I/V inj. Of Sodium Iodide @ 70mg/Kg bw for 7 days.

288. Which organism causes Vibriosis in cattle?

Answer: *Campylobacter foetus*

289. What is the symptom of campylobacteriosis in cattle?

Answer: Abortion is a major complaint between 4th and 7th month of pregnancy.

290. What is the causative organism of Lumpy Jaw?

Answer: *Actinomyces bovis*

291. Name a few organisms that are associated with mastitis in cattle?

Answer: *Staphylococcus spp., Streptococcus spp., Corynebacterium spp., Klebsiella spp., E.coli, Mycobacterium spp., Mycoplasma spp.,*

292. Which breed of cattle are prone to mastitis?

Answer: Cross bred animals are prone to mastitis especially Holstein Friesian crossess.

293. What are the predisposing factors of Mastitis

Answer: a) Ruminal acidosis

b) Impaired udder immunity

c) Improper sanitation

d) Stress on milking animal

e) Drug resistance for recurrent mastitis

294. What happens in per acute mastitis?

Answer: The udder became hard, swelled and inflamed. Watery milk will come and there will be temperature reaction. The animal will be off-fed and in pain

295. Name some test used to detect mastitis in field condition.

Answer: California mastitis test, pH paper test and strip cup test

296. What is Sub Clinical mastitis?

Answer: Sub-clinical mastitis is the term for the condition, which occurs when there are no obvious macroscopic abnormalities in the mammary gland yet bacterial infections are present in the milk.

297. How does sub clinical mastitis hamper the milk quality?

Answer: Milk will have an increased somatic cell count and an alkaline pH. Subclinical mastitis may result in decreased milk fat and SNF.

298. How is the sub clinical mastitis diagnosed? What is the treatment protocol?

Answer: California mastitis test, Bromothymol blue test, Somatic cell count (>1 million cells per ml milk).

Treatment: In positive chronic cases broad spectrum antibiotics may be applied. In newly developed cases Tri Sodium Citrate may be applied for 10-15 days orally @ 10gm daily with feed to maintain blood pH.

299. What is the most widely used Ethno-Veterinary treatment protocol of mastitis?

Answer: Whole Aloe vera leaf – 250 gm, Turmeric powder – 50 gm, Lime – 15 gm. All materials are to be mixed and applied to the udder.

300. How can we distinguish between Udder Oedema and Mastitis?

Answer: In udder edema there will be an edematous swelling over the udder, but there won't be any alterations in the milk's quality. After parturition, udder edema typically starts with agalactia.

301. Which organism causes recurrent mastitis?

Answer: *Staphylococcus aureus*

302. Which organism causes summer mastitis?

Answer: *Acranobacterium pyogenes*

303. State the preventive measures of mastitis?

Answer: a) Animals should be fed during milking

b) Teat dipping should be conducted after milking

c) Calf should not be allowed to fed mother's milk throughout the day

d) Disinfectant should be used to clean herd

e) Proper feeding system should be followed to control ruminal acidosis

304. How mastitis affects in milk business?

Answer: Due to mastitis primarily milk production is reduced by 30-40 per cent. Also, the yield of milk products like Paneer, Cheese reduces drastically.

305. What is the ideal pH of rumen?

Answer: 6.5-7

306. What are the different kinds of ruminal indigestion?

Answer: Simple indigestion, Acid indigestion, Alkaline indigestion

307. What will be ruminal pH for different kinds of indigestion?

Answer: pH in Simple indigestion – 6-7, pH in Acid indigestion 4-5.5, pH in Alkaline indigestion 7.5-8.5

308. How alkaline indigestion takes place?

Answer: Due to a) excessive intake of protein, b) intake of placenta, c) feeding of urea *etc.*, excessive amount of ammonia is produced which can't be utilized by microbes. Excess ammonia is circulated through the portal veins and transformed to urea in the liver. Urea is recycled in the rumen or eliminated through the kidney. Alkaline indigestion results from excessive accumulation of ammonia and urea in the absence of sufficient VFA, which raises the ruminal pH to 7.5–9.5.

309. What is the treatment protocol of Alkaline indigestion?

Answer: 5-10 per cent Acetic acid @5-10 ml/kg body weight orally. 5-10 per cent Acetic acid 200-500 ml orally or intra ruminal.

310. How acid indigestion takes place?

Answer: Gram-positive bacteria proliferate in the rumen when an excessive amount of carbohydrate, such as grain, decomposing silage, kitchen waste, or garbage is suddenly consumed by a ruminant. A significant amount of lactic acid is generated as a result of the quick fermentation of carbohydrates. Ruminal pH is lowered to 5 or less due to the accumulation of lactic acid and initially produced VFA in the rumen. The condition developed is ruminal indigestion or ruminal acidosis.

311. What is the treatment protocol for acid indigestion?

Answer: Sodium bicarbonate 2.5 – 5 per cent solution 500 ml to 1 lit through I/V route. Followed by isotonic 1.3 per cent NaHCO3 @ 150 ml/kg body weight may be given. Straw should be given in this situation. Also, Penicillin 50-100 Lakh may be given.

312. What are the causative organisms of Theileriosis, Babesiosis, Anaplasmosis and Trypanosomiasis?

Answer: Babesiosis– *Babesia bigemina, Babesia bovis*

Theileriosis – *Theileria annulata, Theileria parva*

Trypanosomiasis - *Trypanosoma evansi*

Anaplasmosis – *Anaplasma marginale*

313. State the symptoms and treatment of Babesiosis.

Answer: Haemoglobinurea, high rise of temperature, anorexia and severe weakness.

Drug of choice – a) Diminazine aceturate @3.5 mg per kg body weight I/M

b) Imidocarb @ 1 mg per kg body weight S/C

314. State the symptoms and treatment of Theileriosis.

Answer: Engorgement of superficial lymph node, initially 106°F temperature followed by 104°F temperature, anorexia, jaundice.

Drug of choice: Buparvoquone @ 2.5 mg per kg body weight I/M.

315. Differentiate between duck plague and duck cholera

Answer: Duck plague or duck viral enteritis is a viral disease caused by herpes virus whereas Duck Cholera or duck pasteurellosis is a bacterial disease caused by *Pasteurella multocida*.

316. Why F strain is used for Ranikhet vaccine preparation?

Answer: F strain is a lentogenic strain or low virulence strain so vaccine prepared from this strain have little adverse effect.

317. How is the Ranikhet disease (F1 strain) vaccine administered to flock?

Answer: Intra-nasal or Intra-ocular. For mass vaccination it is administered through cold drinking water or by aerosol spray.

318. What is lapinization? Name a lapinized vaccine.

Answer: Lapinization means the serial passage of a virus through rabbits to attenuate it.

Example: Classical swine fever vaccine prepared from Hog cholera virus LOM strain.

319. Name a polyvalent tissue culture vaccine

Answer: FMD vaccine

320. Give an example of oil adjuvant vaccine

Answer: Haemorrhagic Septicaemia vaccine.

321. Which strain of vaccine is used in Brucella CP program in India?

Answer: S19 strain of Brucella abortus

322. Name a mycoplasmal disease which can be prevented by vaccination.

Answer: CCPP (Contagious Caprine Pleuro-Pneumonia) and CBPP (Contagious Bovine Pleuro-Pneumonia.

323. What is lumpy skin disease (LSD)?

Answer: Lumpy skin disease (LSD) is caused by lumpy skin disease virus (LSDV), a virus from the family *Poxviridae*, genus *Capripoxvirus*. Sheep pox virus and goat pox virus are the two other virus species in this genus.

324. Which domestic animals may be affected by LSD?

Answer: LSD mainly affects cattle, although water buffalo can be affected. In general, crossbred cattle and exotic cattle (*Bos taurus*) are more vulnerable than native zebu cattle (*Bos indicus*). LSD has been seen in wild ruminants, but it is not transmitted to people.

325. When and where was LSD first reported in India and West Bengal?

Answer: In India – August 2019 in Odisha

In West Bengal –September 2019

326. How LSD transmits?

Answer: LSD is primarily spread via vectors. The ability to propagate the LSD virus has been established by biting insects, including the common stable fly (*Stomoxys calcitrans*), the mosquito (*Aedes aegypti*), and various tick species of the *Rhipicephalus* and *Amblyomma* spp. Saliva, milk, semen, necrotic tissue, nasal secretions, and vaginal secretions from an infected animals acts as contaminants by which the LSD virus can spread. The mechanical transmission of the LSD virus can be facilitated by contaminated food, clothing, equipment, feeders, waterers, syringes, and needles (including artificial insemination devices).

327. State the morbidity and mortality losses caused by LSD.

Answer: Morbidity varies according to the nature of the disease outbreak and the herd's level of immunity. An outbreak can initially infect between 10 and 20 percent of animals. Calves older than one month can have a morbidity of up to 40 per cent.

328. State the clinical signs and symptoms of LSD.

Answer: Mild fever for two to three days follows the development of stiff, spherical cutaneous nodules (2 to 5 cm in diameter) on the skin all over the body. These elevated, firm, spherical, confined nodules affect the skin, subcutaneous tissue, and occasionally the muscles.

Emaciation, swollen lymph nodes, oedema of the limbs, decreased milk production, abortion, infertility, and occasionally death are among the symptoms that might occur.

329. What are the long-term side effects of LSD?

Answer:

- Pneumonia may be caused by the virus itself or secondary bacterial infections
- Mastitis

☆ Permanent or temporary infertility in bulls

☆ Abortion or anestrus lasting for several months

330. State the control measures of LSD.

Answer:

a) Control of animal mobility: All animal movement into and out of the affected region should be prohibited.

b) Restrictions of human movement - Animal handlers and people dealing with the affected animals should be advised to keep out of the healthy animals.

c) Vector control - Insecticides, repellents, and other chemical agents should be used to manage the vector population (ticks, flies, mosquitoes, and fleas) on the premises and on animals.

d) Use of sodium hypochlorite (2–3 per cent) solution for cleaning and disinfecting purposes.

331. What vaccine may be applied to control LSD?

Answer: Cattle and buffaloes should be vaccinated with Goat pox - GTPV vaccine (Uttarkashi strain) among all animals above 4 months of age through S/C route.

332. What is the treatment protocol of LSD?

Answer: Symptomatic care, including the management of any secondary infections, must be provided and the infected animal should be isolated.

a) Using anti-inflammatory medications to treat the inflammatory conditions, preferably without steroids

b) Using antihistamine medications or preparations to treat allergic symptoms

c) Antibiotics may also be used to treat secondary bacterial infections such respiratory and skin diseases. Streptopenicillin, Ceftriaxone, Ceftiofur, and Enrofloxacin can be administered properly in recommended dose and route. Oral treatment with 0.1 per cent Methylene Blue solution often bear good result.

333. Write the treatment protocol of LSD by using Methylene Blue.

Answer: Oral treatment with 0.1 per cent Methylene Blue (MB) solution (1 gram of MB powder in 1 liter of water) may be considered.

Following dosage may be attempted:

☆ Adult cows (of approximately 350 Kg body weight): 300 ml at 8 hourly intervals (Thrice in a day) for 4 days.

☆ Calf: Give approx half dose

MB solution/preparations may also be used topically by spray.

334. Which sample to be collected for laboratory diagnosis of LSD?

Answer:

a) Scabs are a great source of sample material since they are simple to harvest, don't need to be sedated or given anesthesia, and have high viral concentrations that can be transported for long distances while surviving well in a variety of climates. There should be a combined sample taken from three separate locations on the animal.

b) Saliva or nasal swabs can be collected using sterile swabs.

c) Blood for serum samples must be collected without anticoagulant.

335. Name the different organisms that cause abortion in cattle in different trimester.

Answer: Bovine Viral Diarrhoea: The Togaviridae family of pestiviruses is the cause. Infertility may occur prior to insemination and embryonic mortality comes from infection during the first 40 days of pregnancy.If the foetus survives from the infection, it leads to the birth of persistently infected calves between 40 and 125 days of pregnancy. Congenital CNS abnormalities, such as cerebellar hypoplasia, hydrocephalus, *etc.*, can be caused by foetal infection during the organogenesis phase (100–150 days).BVD may result in abortion after 125 days of pregnancy.

Brucellosis: Caused by *Brucella abortus*. Brucellosis causes abortions in the second half of gestation (usually by 7 months).

Campylobacteriosis: Caused by *Campylobacter jejuni* and *Campylobacter foetus foetus*. By ingestion and subsequent hematogenous transmission organisms reach to the placenta. *C foetus foetus* and *C jejuni* are contagious. Both have infrequent abortion-causing effects, generally in the second half of pregnancy.

Infectious bovine rhinotracheitis (IBR): Bovine herpes virus I is responsible. The virus spreads to the placenta, where it causes placentitis. After the foetus acquires the infection, it dies within 24 hours. While abortions can happen at any moment but often start around four months.

Leptospirosis: Caused by the seven serotypes of *Leptospira interrogans*. Abortions are typically caused by *Leptospira* serovars Grippotyphosa, Pomona, Canicola, and Icterohaemorrhagiae in the third trimester, 2–6 weeks following maternal infection.

Listeriosis: *Listeria monocytogenes* causes the disease. Abortions are typically sporadic and can happen at any stage of pregnancy. The mother may experience fever and anorexia before the abortion, and retained placenta is frequently seen. Abortion typically occurs from four months onward during pregnancy.

Mycotic abortion: Caused by *Aspergillus* sp. It is an important factor contributing to sporadic bovine abortion. Abortions happen after four months of pregnancy and are most common in the winter.

336. Name the different organisms that cause abortion in sheep.

Answer:

Bluetongue: It results in foetal mummification, stillbirth, abortion, and congenital brain defects in lambs.

Enzootic Abortion of Ewes: Late-term abortions, stillbirths, and weak lambs are characteristics of the *Chlamydophila abortus* infection. Regardless of when infection starts, abortions happen within the final 2-3 weeks of pregnancy.

Brucellosis: Infectious epididymitis in rams is caused by *Brucella ovis*. In addition to stillbirths, late-term abortions and the delivery of poor lambs found in eves. Brucellosis results in infertility too.

337. Name the different organisms that cause abortion in goats.

Answer:

Caprine herpesvirus 1: It frequently results in late-term abortion outbreaks that are unrelated to other clinical symptoms.

Brucellosis: The most important organism involved in abortion is *Brucella melitensis*. Mastitis and lameness are possible side effects of abortion, which is most common in the fourth month.

Coxiella burnetii: It is a significant contributor to caprine abortion. The most frequent are late-term abortions, stillbirths *etc.*

Listeriosis: *Listeria monocytogenes* is a common pathogen in goats and causes sporadic abortion and severe metritis after abortion.

338. Name the different organisms that cause abortion in pigs.

Answer: Brucellosis: The causing agent is *Brucella suis*, and endometritis and foetal infection are likely responsible for the abortion.

Classical swine fever (Hog Cholera): Caused by pestivirus and causes serious maternal illness and abortion.

Leptospirosis: *Leptospira interrogans* (especially serovar Pomona) is a major cause of reproductive failure in swine causes infertility, abortion, stillbirths *etc.*

339. What is milk fever?

Answer: Milk fever is a metabolic disorder marked by hypocalcaemia, alterations in neuromuscular tone, recumbency, circulatory collapse, and eventually a loss of consciousness.

340. What is the body temperature of cow in milk fever?

Answer: Temperature generally remains subnormal.

341. When milk fever occurs?

Answer: Within 3 to 7 days of parturition.

342. Which lactations are most vulnerable to Milk fever?

Answer: Cows in their 3rd lactation and older, aged 5 to 10 years are most vulnerable.

343. What is the seasonal effect in milk fever?

Answer: It is more common in the winter than in the summer.

344. What are the causes of milk fever?

Answer: Normal animals maintain calcium homeostasis at about 9–10 mg/dl, but a milk fever-affected cow's blood calcium level drops to 5–2.5 mg/dl. Milk fever develops as a result of high calcium loss in the milk immediately following parturition.

Factor described below:

The calcium content of colostrum is 12–13 times higher than that of blood. Milk fever is caused by an excessive loss of calcium in the colostrum that exceeds the intestine's ability to absorb calcium and bones' ability to restore the same.

345. Which hormone is associated with Milk fever?

Answer: Parathormone, Calcitonin, Estrogen and Vit D3 are related to milk fever.

346. How Parathormone is related to milk fever?

Answer: Consuming calcium during the dry season has an impact on this issue. Because excessive calcium depresses the activity of "PTH" and its gland, a high calcium intake (above 100–125 g/cow/day) during the dry period has the tendency to make the issue worse. In contrast, feeding low calcium (8 g/day/450 kg body weight) and high phosphorus during the dry period stimulates "PTH" activity and prepares the gland for the enhanced activity necessary at parturition.

347. Why Vit D_3 is called as hormone?

Answer: Cholecalciferol, or vitamin D_3, is a crucial element in milk fever. The liver and kidney enzymes convert this vitamin D_3 first into 25-hydroxy cholecalciferol and then 1,25-dihydroxy cholecalciferol, respectively. "PTH" has an impact on the entire process. The activated form of vitamin D_3, 1-25 dihydroxy cholecalciferol, acts on gut cells to aid in calcium absorption from the intestine and calcium resorption from bone to keep the blood's calcium levels balanced positively. Because of these physiochemical characteristics, vitamin D_3 is now referred to be a hormone.

348. What is the calcium to phosphorus ratio in blood?

Answer: 2.3:1

349. What is milk fever syndrome or milk fever complex?

Answer: The term "milk fever syndrome" or "milk fever complex" is used to describe the condition when the milk fever is accompanied by hypocalcaemia, hypophosphataemia, and hypomagnesaemia.

350. What are the other diseases caused due to hypocalcaemia?

Answer: In addition to milk fever, dystocia, uterine prolapse, retained placenta (ROP), metritis, abomasal displacement, and mastitis can all be caused by hypocalcemia.

351. Describe the stages of milk fever.

Answer:

Stage 1

- Cows are mobile and standing, yet they exhibit reactivity and hyperactivity.
- They may exhibit ear twitching, head bobbing, triceps- and flank-tremors, and minor ataxia.
- Cows may bellow, shuffle their back feet, appear to be uncomfortable.

Stage 2:

- Due to extreme paresthesia to this stage where cows are unable to stand.
- To sustain sternal recumbency, they do possess sufficient muscular control.
- They often have an obtunded appearance, are anorexic, have a dry muzzle, a low body temperature, and cold extremities.
- Due to compromised cardiac contractility, auscultation demonstrates tachycardia and decreased intensity of heart sounds.
- There are few peripheral pulses.

- ☆ Bloating, inability to urinate, and loss of anal sphincter tone are symptoms of smooth muscle paralysis, which causes gastrointestinal stasis.
- ☆ On rectal examination, a distended bladder may indicate an inability to urinate.
- ☆ A cow's head will frequently tuck into its sides.
- ☆ Due to the asymmetry of the cervical vertebrae, if the cow can extend its head, the neck may have an S-shaped curvature.

Stage 3:

- ☆ With parturient paresis gradually lose awareness until they enter a state of coma.
- ☆ They can only rest flat on their sides and cannot sustain sternal recumbency.
- ☆ They can have considerable bloat, have extremely flaccid muscles, and possibly be unresponsive to stimulation.
- ☆ Heart rate can increase to 120 bpm as cardiac output declines, and peripheral pulses may become undetected.
- ☆ Cows at stage 3 may only survive a short time if untreated.

352. State the line of treatment for milk fever.

Answer:

- ☆ Oral calcium supplementation for standing cows

  The standing animals can be treated with an oral calcium gel supplement since it quickly reaches the bloodstream and has a low risk of hypocalcemia rebound. A typical oral dose of calcium contains 40–55 g of elemental calcium.

- ☆ Intravenous calcium infusion for recumbent cows

  Cows who are recumbent and have stage 2 or stage 3 hypocalcemia require intravenous calcium infusion. An adult dairy cow will typically get 450 mL of a 20 per cent calcium boro-gluconate solution as therapy. This common procedure delivers 9–10 g of elemental calcium, which is enough to restore calcium.

  The most effective intravenous treatment for parturient paresis is calcium boro-gluconate alone. The calcium boro-gluconate solution should always be infused slowly.

  The I/M therapy should be combined with the addition of vitamin D3.

353. Why is calcium borogluconate used instead of using calcium gluconate to treat a milk fever case?

Answer: To solubilize the calcium gluconate and stabilise the solution, boric acid is added to the calcium gluconate solution.

354. How Ketosis takes place in ruminant? What are the predisposing factors of Ketosis?

Answer: Starvation causes a significant deficiency of carbohydrates in the liver cells of ruminant. It causes fat molecules to undergo beta oxidation, which creates acetone and ketone bodies. It causes ketoacidosis, ketonuria, and ketolactia. The condition is known as ketosis.

The following are the predisposing factors of Ketosis:

a) Lack of nutritive feed
b) Adreno cortisol insufficiency
c) Hypothyroidism
d) Hepatic insufficiency
e) Loss of appetite due to disease
f) Deficiency of cobalt

355. Write the treatment protocol of Ketosis.

Answer: 500-800 ml of 40-50 per cent solution of glucose (dextrose) should be given I/V at once.

225 mg glycerin may be offered orally BD. Dexamethasone or Betamethasone are given up to 30 mg once.

356. Name few Ketone bodies.

Answer: Aceto-acetic acid, beta-hydroxybutyric acid *etc.*

357. Which animals are susceptible to Ketosis?

Answer: Occurs mostly in milking animals. Cattle, buffalo and ewe suffer from this condition.

358. Why do high yielding cattle mostly suffer from Ketosis?

Answer: Because all high-yielding cows in the early lactation remain in negative energy balance and high-yielding cattle typically suffer at any point during the lactation period.

359. In which lactation Ketosis is common?

Answer: In the third lactation or later, ketosis occurs more frequently. Occasionally, dry cows in their late stages of pregnancy may exhibit this.

360. What is primary ketosis?

Answer: Underfeeding or starvation cause ketosis. Typically, it happens from the first week to eight weeks after calving. Primary ketosis results from a persistent imbalance in the metabolism of fats and carbohydrates caused by fasting or underfeeding.

361. What is secondary ketosis?

Answer: When animals are offered food during the course of a sickness, but they refuse it because of inappetence, this syndrome develops. This leads to an imbalance in the levels of carbohydrates and lipids.

362. What is Ketogenic ketosis?

Answer: The digestive form of ketosis is known as ketogenic ketosis.

363. How does the alimentary or digestive form of ketosis occur?

Answer: Microbial fermentation of carbohydrates produces VFA in the form of acetic acid, propionic acid, and butyric acid. Propionic acid is glucogenic, butyric acid and acetic acid are ketogenic. To sustain excellent health, these two groups of acids should be produced in a ratio of roughly 4:1. Ketosis may occur if the diet contains excessive amount of ketogenic ingredients, such as silage, hay, *etc.* Silage is more ketogenic than hay, and silage made from succulent materials may be more ketogenic than other types of silages due to the availability of a larger quantity of preformed butyric acid. This form of ketosis is called as digestive or alimentary ketosis.

364. How Ketosis develops?

Answer: Fatty acids turn into ketones rather than glucose when CoA is absent or unavailable. Acetic acid, propionic acid, and butyric acid are produced from carbohydrates. Activated acetate is produced through the reaction of acetic acid and butyric acid. Fatty acids are transformed into energy via the TCA cycle because oxalo-acetate is readily available. Additionally, the activated acetate is transformed into aceto-acidic acid and beta-hydroxybutyric acid when oxalo-acetate is not present. Major Ketone bodies in an animal's body include aceto-acidic acid and B-hydroxybutyric acid.

365. In a high yielding cow how much body fat and body protein are drained out during milk production daily?

Answer: A cow with a daily capacity of 20–40 litres of milk expels 1-2 kg of body fat and 0.6–1 kg of body protein during milk production.

366. What is the relationship of liver with ketosis?

Answer: The liver houses the glycogen. Lactic acid is converted into glycogen by hepatic cells, and then glucose is produced from glycogen. Hypoglycemia, however, is a characteristic of hepatic inactivity and results in ketosis.

367. How cobalt is related with ketosis?

Answer: Cobalt deficiency prevents the synthesis of Vitamin B12 (cyanocobalamin), which prevents the production of epinephrine. Lack of epinephrine prevents gluconeogenesis, which results in hypoglycemia and ketosis.

368. What are the clinical findings in digestive form of ketosis?

Answer:

- A sudden loss of body weight;
- A decrease in hunger over a period of two to four days;
- A sharp reduction in milk output;
- Cows can appear "woody" due to apparent wasting and the absence of subcutaneous lipids.
- The eyes become dull, typically the head is held low, though occasionally the cow may adopt a "star-gazing" posture;
- The stool is dry and coated with mucus;
- There may be subnormal temperature caused by hypoglycaemia;
- Ruminal movements may be lowered in amplitude and rate;
- Ruminal motions may also be decreased in frequency.
- A few affected animals may die if untreated;
- Distinctive ketone body odour (sweet to vinegary smell) is visible on the breath and in milk.

369. What is the nervous form of ketosis?

Answer: As a result of hypoglycemia, the type of ketosis manifests anxious symptoms. The symptoms include circling movement, crossing of the legs, pressing the head into the feeding dish or leaning into it, blindness, aimless wandering, and vigorous licking of inanimate objects and skin. If you pinch the animal, it bellows. The gait is stumbling, and there could be some mild tremor and tetany. The anxious symptoms can return after an eight- to twelve-hour break and last for one to two hours.

370. What is Ketolactia?

Answer: If ketone bodies are present in milk, it will be termed as Ketolactia.

371. What will be the level of ketone bodies in milk and urine during Ketosis?

Answer: In milk – 40 mg/dl and in urine – 500-1000 mg/dl.

372. What changes will be seen in serum calcium and magnesium levels during ketosis?

Answer: Serum calcium and magnesium level will fall due to ketosis.

373. State the treatment protocol of Ketosis.

Answer:

- Glycerine may be given orally @ 225 mg BD for 3 – 5 days
- Sodium propionate may be given orally @ 100 – 200 gm daily for 3 – 5 days

- ☆ Dextrose 25 per cent solution may be given I/V @ 500 ml daily for 3 – 5 days
- ☆ Betamethasone and dexamethasone can be given upto 30 mg I/m.
- ☆ Prednisolone acetate may be given @ 10 ml I/m
- ☆ Vit. B1, B6, B12 should be given I/m or I/v for 3 – 5 days

374. What is Post parturient hemoglobinuria?

Answer: Post-parturient hemoglobinuria is a rare illness that can occur anywhere in the world. It typically strikes individual high-yielding dairy cows at the start of lactation. Acute intravascular hemolysis that frequently results in hemoglobinuria and can cause life-threatening anaemia are its defining features.

375. What are the causes of Post parturient hemoglobinuria?

Answer: Phosphorus depletion or hypophosphatemia, copper deficiency, and possibly hemolyzing chemicals found in some feeds have all been implicated as potential causes or predisposing factors, while the actual reason remains unknown.

376. What is hypomagnesemic tetany?

Answer: The complicated metabolic problem known as hypomagnesemic tetany causes hyperexcitability, muscle spasms, seizures, respiratory difficulty, collapse, and death. It is characterized by hypomagnesemia and a decreased concentration of magnesium in the CSF.

377. How can we classify the Hypomagnesemic tetany?

Answer: According to aetiology it can be classified as follows:

- ☆ Lactation tetany: This is brought on by consuming an excessive amount of green grass while also consuming an excessive amount of milk. It is always related to lactation.
- ☆ Grass tetany: It happens in animals kept on recently grown, green grass that are magnesium deficient.
- ☆ Milk tetany: may be seen in calves who are given only milk, which is often referred to as "whole milk tetany." Magnesium is insufficient in milk.
- ☆ Transit tetany:(Transport tetany) It frequently happens in late pregnancy and after a lengthy journey in cows and ewes. It is characterised by unconsciousness, gastrointestinal stasis, and recumbency.
- ☆ Winter tetany: Hypo-magnesaemia is more common in the winter since pastures are less developed and still have low magnesium contents.

378. What is the normal magnesium level in cattle blood?

Answer: 2.3 mg/dl

379. State the clinical findings of Hypomagnesemic tetany.

Answer: Affected cows have severe paddling seizures with chewing of the jaws, frothy salivation, fluttering of the eyelids, and nystagmus in the most severe form of hypomagnesemic tetany. Short-interval recurrences of seizures are possible, and death typically happens within a few hours.

380. State the line of treatment of Hypomagnesemic tetany.

Answer: Calcium and Magnesium combination should be administered I/V to tackle the situation. Calcium Magnesium borogluconate(Inj. Mifex) is recommended @ 250 ml to 450 ml I/V in acute cases.

381. State the vaccination schedule of Canine

Answer:

Age of Puppy	*Vaccine*	*Route of Inoculation*	*Revaccination*
4-6 weeks	Puppy DP (Distemper and Parvo)	S/C	
8-9 weeks	DHPPi-L – 1(CD, ICH, Parvo, Para Influenza, Leptospira)	S/C	
12 weeks	DHPPi-L – 2	S/C	Revaccinated annually
15-16 weeks	Rabies	1 ml S/C	Revaccinated annually

382. Describe the vaccination schedule for Broiler, Backyard Poultry bird and Commercial layer in chicken and duck

Answer: Following Standard vaccine schedule practiced for poultry in general, but it may vary in different area depends on disease prevalence for particular area.

Vaccination Schedule for Broiler

Age	*Vaccine*	*Route of Administration*
1st Day	IB live vaccine (optional)	I/O or I/N
5-7th day	Ranikhet Disease/ND live vaccine	I/O or I/N
12th day	IBD live Vaccine	I/O or I/N
21st day	Ranikhet Disease/ND live vaccine (La sota strain)	Drinking water

Vaccination schedule for Backyard poultry

Age	*Vaccine*	*Type*	*Diluents used*	*Route*
1st day	Marek's disease vaccine (optional)	Freeze dried live	NSS/Distilled water	0.2ml S/C
5-7th day	Ranikhet Disease/ND live vaccine	Freeze dried live	NSS/Distilled water	I/O or I/N
14th day	IBD live Vaccine	Freeze dried live	NSS/Distilled water	I/O or I/N
24th day	IBD live Vaccine	Freeze dried live		Drinking water
35th day	Ranikhet Disease/ND live vaccine (La sota starin)	do		Drinking water
42nd day	Fowl Pox vaccine (CEVL or PPCEVL)	Freeze dried live	Chilled 50 per cent buffered glycerol saline or NSS/ Distilled water	Feather follicle or wing webI/M (NSS/ Distilled water)
56th day	Ranikhet Disease/ND live vaccine (La sota strain)	Freeze dried live		Drinking water
63rd day	Deworming			
70th Day	R2B live vaccine	Freeze dried live	NSS/Distilled water	0.2 ml I/M inj
R2B live vaccine or ND live vaccine may be repeated in every one-month interval				

Vaccination Schedule for Duck

Age	*Vaccine*	*Type*	*Diluents Used*	*Route*
1st dose. 30th day. Repeat after one month, then revaccinate at every 6 months	Duck Cholera	Inactivated, adjuvanated		1 ml S/C
1st dose: 45th day. Repeat after 6 months, then once in a year	Duck Plague	Freeze dried live	NSS/ Distilled water	I/O or I/N

Vaccination Schedule for Commercial Layer

Age	*Vaccine*	*Type*	*Diluents used*	*Route*
0 day	IB live vaccine	Freeze dried live	NSS/Distilled water	I/O or I/N Beak dipping
0 day	Marek's (VVMD) vaccine	Freeze dried live	NSS/Distilled water	0.2ml S/C
5th day	Ranikhet Disease -ND live vaccine	Freeze dried live	NSS/Distilled water	I/O or I/N
5th day	(ND+IBD) combined killed vaccine	Killed vaccine		0.2ml S/C
9th day	Touching			
12th day	IBD live Vaccine	Freeze dried live	NSS/Distilled water	I/O or I/N
21st day	IB live vaccine	Freeze dried live	NSS/Distilled water	I/O or I/N
24th day	IBD live Vaccine	Freeze dried live		Drinking water
30th day	Ranikhet Disease/ND live vaccine (La sota strain)	Freeze dried live		Drinking water
42nd day	Fowl Pox vaccine (CEVL or PPCEVL)	Freeze dried live	Chilled 50 per cent buffered glycerol saline	Feather follicle Or wing web, 0.2 ml
49th day	Fowl Coryza – Killed vaccine	Killed		0.5 ml I/M
56th day	Ranikhet Disease/ND live vaccine (La sota strain)	Freeze dried live		Drinking water
63rd day	Deworming			
70th day	R2B live vaccine	Freeze dried live	NSS/Distilled water	0.2 ml I/M inj.
84th day	(ND+IB) combined live vaccine	Freeze dried live		Drinking water
91st day	Fowl pox vaccine			
98th day	Fowl Coryza – Killed vaccine	Killed vaccine		0.5 ml I/M
110th day	(ND+IB) combined killed vaccine	Killed vaccine		0.5m I/M
ND live vaccine may be repeated in every one-month interval				

383. State the vaccination schedule of Sheep and Goat.

Answer:

Vaccine	*Recommended Diluent*	*Dose and Route of Inoculation*	*Periodicity of Vaccination*
Cell culture Freeze dried Goat Pox Live vaccine	100 ml Chilled PBS	1 ml S/C	1st dose at 12 weeks of age and revaccinated annually
Cell culture Freeze dried PPR Live vaccine	100 ml Chilled NSS	1 ml S/C	1st dose at 16 weeks of age and revaccinated after 3 years

384. State the vaccination schedule of Pig.

Answer:

Vaccine	*Recommended Diluent*	*Dose and Route of Inoculation*	*Periodicity of Vaccination*
Swine fever (lapinized) Freeze dried Live vaccine	5 ml Chilled NSS	1 ml S/C	1st dose at 8 to 9 weeks of age and revaccinated annually

385. Vaccination schedule for cattle and buffalo in field condition.

Answer:

Disease	*Vaccine*	*Time of Vaccine*	*Immunity*	*Dose*	*Remarks*
FMD	Oil adjuvant (BioFMD-OIL vaccine in recent FMDCP Programme	Any cattle beyond 6 months of age	One season	2 ml I/M	Generally, in Oct-Nov
Bruce-llosis	S19 (Live) strain in BrucellaCP Programme	4-8 months of age only female calves	Life long	2 ml S/C	Only once in lifetime
HS	HS vaccine (inactivated adjuvanated)	3rd to 6th month of age, Revaccination at every 6 months interval	Six months	5 ml S/C	In endemic areas

Disease	*Vaccine*	*Time of Vaccine*	*Immunity*	*Dose*	*Remarks*
BQ	BQ vaccine (inactivated adjuvanated)	3rd to 6th month of age, Repeat after 4 weeks and then yearly vaccination	One year	5 ml S/C	In endemic areas
Anthrax	Anthrax Spore Vaccine (Live)	3rd to 5th month of age. Yearly revaccination	One year	1 ml S/C	In endemic areas

386. What is the deworming schedule commonly practiced for cattle, buffalo, sheep and goat in field condition?

Answer: First deworming should be done at the age of one month Then animals should be dewormed at every month with broad spectrum anthelmentics up to six months of age.

Periodic deworming after the age of six months should be carried out every three months interval or as and when required on the basis of clinical manifestation or stool examination.

387. What is the deworming schedule commonly practiced for dog and cat?

Answer: The best method to prevent an infestation for both ourselves and our dogs is to follow a comprehensive deworming routine. Deworming should be done on puppies and kittens every two weeks until they are 3 months old, then once per month until they are 6 months of age. Following that, deworming of dog/cat four times a year is adequate.

388. Why it is advisable to deworm at least seven days before vaccination?

Answer: Parasitic load in animal lowers the immunity of animal. Vaccination in worm loaded animal reduces antibody response to vaccine. Therefore deworming before vaccination is always advisable for proper immune response to vaccination and also to get the desired immunity of the animal.

389. What are the different types of fluids used intravenously in veterinary field and state the compositions of those fluids?

Answer:

Sl.No.	*Name*	*Presentation*	*Composition*
1	Normal Saline	500 ml,1 Lit	Sodium Chloride – 0.9 per cent
2	DNS (Dextrose Normal Saline)	500 ml	Sodium Chloride – 0.9 per cent Dextrose – 5 per cent
3	D5	500 ml	Dextrose – 5 per cent
4	D10	500 ml	Dextrose – 10 per cent

Sl.No.	*Name*	*Presentation*	*Composition*
5	D25	500 ml	Dextrose – 25 per cent
6	Dextrose with multiple electrolyte (Rinctose or Intalyte)	500 ml,1 Lit	Dextrose – 20 per cent Sodium Chloride – 0.6 per cent Potassium Chloride - 0.04 per cent Calcium chloride – 0.027 per cent Sodium lactate – 0.312 per cent
7	Ringer Lactate	500 ml	Sodium Chloride – 0.6 per cent Potassium Chloride - 0.04 per cent Calcium chloride – 0.027 per cent Sodium lactate – 0.32 per cent
8	Calcium Borogluconate (Calborol)	450 ml	Calcium Gluconate – 1.86 per cent Proportion of Boric Acid to Calcium 2.26 to 1 Chlorocresol – 0.1 per cent
9	Calcium Magnesium Borogluconate (Mifex)	450 ml	Calcium gluconate – 1.86 per cent Proportion of Boric acid to Calcium 2.26 to 1 Magnesium hypophosphite – 5 per cent Dextrose – 20 per cent Chlorocresol – 0.1 per cent

390. What is the difference between A1 and A2 milk?

Answer: A1 and A2 are two genetic types of the beta-casein milk protein. Two distinct milk protein types, A1 and A2, can be found in cow's milk. A single amino acid change in the beta-casein protein, which accounts for around 30 per cent of cow milk protein composition, distinguishes milk from A1 to A2. The beta-casein protein in A1 milk has the amino acid histidine at position 67, whereas the amino acid proline is present in A2 milk. The different amino acid sequences have an impact on how the protein is digested.

391. What are A1 and A2 cows?

Answer: A1 cows are those that generate both A1 and A2 beta casein proteins, whereas A2 cows are those that solely produce A2 beta casein.

392. Give examples of A1 and A2 cows.

Answer: A1 cow breeds are Jersy, Holstein Friesian, Ayrshire, and British Short horn. A2 cows are Gir, Red Sindhi, Sahiwal, Kankrej, *etc.*

393. Is there any harmful effect of A1 milk in human health?

Answer: A1 beta-casein and the peptide Beta-casomorphin 7 (BCM-7) may be related to diabetes, heart disease, autism, and SIDS, according to a few studies. Still, the findings are contradictory, and more study is required.

394. What are the different methods of physical examination of animals?

Answer: a) Inspection, b) Palpation, c) Percussion, d) Auscultation

395. What is percussion?

Answer: In a physical examination, percussion is the technique of tapping various body parts with the fingers, hands, or small instruments. It is done to determine:

- ✰ The shape, texture, and borders of bodily organs
- ✰ The existence or absence of fluid in certain bodily regions
- ✰ A sound similar to playing a drum is produced when a body part is beaten
- ✰ A physical component or organ's sound indicates the sort of tissue that exists there.
- ✰ Since air fills the lungs, percussion makes them sound empty.
- ✰ Solid organs including the liver and bones, joints, and other bones sound solid.
- ✰ The abdomen makes a hollow organ-like sound that could be filled with air, liquid, or substances.

396. What is tactile percussion?

Answer: In this modified type of percussion, palpation and percussion are carried out simultaneously to determine the consistency and boundaries of deeply-located organs. With this technique, a pregnancy diagnosis may be made.

397. What is Ballottement?

Answer: The method of pregnancy diagnosis through Tactile percussion is known as Ballottement.

398. What is the use of a Stethoscope?

Answer: A medical tool called a stethoscope is used for auscultation, or listening to an animal's or body's internal sounds. A stethoscope can be used to hear the heartbeat, lungs, or intestines as well as the blood flowing via arteries and veins.

399. What is fever?

Answer: Any type of rise in body temperature is referred to or described as having a "fever." Animals typically experience fever as a response to the noxious and frequently contagious compounds known as pyrogens. Pyrogen disrupts the body's system for controlling body temperature, which raises it whatever the ambient temperature.

400. Classify fever etiologically and clinically.

Answer:

Etiologically:

a) Protein fever: Due to administration of foreign protein
b) Salt fever: Due to injection of hypertonic solution
c) Neurogenic fever: Due to damage of brain cells
d) Transitory fever: Due to excessive dehydration
e) Drug fever: Due to drug interaction
f) Idiopathic fever: Fever due to specific virus or bacterial agent
g) Symptomatic fever: Due to localized infections or trauma

Clinically:

a) Acute fever: Sudden sharp rise of body temperature to 104°F or above.
b) Subacute fever: Temperature remains within 103°F to 104°F
c) Chronic fever: Due to some chronic disease temperature persists within 102°F to 103°F for a prolong time.

401. What is Jugular pulsation?

Answer: Jugular pulse refers to the jugular vein's pulse. Jugular pulses can be separated into positive and negative jugular pulses.

402. What is positive Jugular pulsation and when is it observed?

Answer: A real pulse wave that extends from the mandibular angle to the shoulder area is indicated by a positive jugular pulse. Jugular veins are still completely engorged with blood. It gets unusually full and tense. These effects are brought on by traumatic pericarditis and tricuspid valve dysfunction. Blood flows back into the jugular vein. Brisket oedema frequently coexists with a positive jugular pulse.

403. What is negative Jugular pulsation?

Answer: When blood cannot enter the right atrium and eventually backflow occurs in the jugular vein, a negative jugular pulse is observed in cattle. This may be seen in tricuspid valve stenosis.

404. Different Characteristic Postures related to a specific condition

Postures	*Disease/Disorder*
Arching of back with the limb tucked under the body	TRP, Pyelonephritis(Mild abdominal pain)
Downward arching of back and 'Saw horse' straddling of legs	Severe abdominal pain
Prolonged standing in cattle and buffaloes	Pneumonia, pleurisy and pericarditis
Lateral deviation of head	Listeriosis and Gid
A cow or buffalo adopting frog like posture	Bilateral hip dislocation
A cow or buffalo sitting on sternum and the head resting on the flank	Milk fever
Listening attitude in sheep and goat	Early stages of pregnancy toxemia and scrapie
Frog like posture in sheep and goat	Parturient hypocalcaemia
A horse shifting its weight from one limb to another	Laminits, osteodystrophia fibrosa
A horse adopting dog sitting posture associated with rolling and kicking at belly	Acute gastric dilatation
Typical rigid/wooden horse posture	Tetanus
Male dog urinating like bitch	Cystitis, Urolithiasis
A dog showing upward arching of its back (Kyphosis)	Acute nephritis

405. Describe in details about the collection, preservation and dispatch of different samples for diagnosis of different diseases in field condition.

Answer:

COLLECTION, PRESERVATION AND DESPATCH OF SAMPLES

It is a fundamental principle for any laboratory test procedure that the results depend on the quality of the samples. The results of the test may be negative if the specimen has not been properly collected, labelled, and stored prior to and during the test process. So, to obtain quick and correct results, we should maintain the following during the sending of samples.

The following points should be considered during collection of samples for laboratory testing.

a) All materials collected should be accompanied with full history *viz* clinical signs, course of the disease, morbidity, mortality in species affected, tentative diagnosis *etc.*

b) The materials from ailing animals should be collected at height of body temperature and clinical signs and when the clinical sings of the disease is prominent in animal.

c) For serological diagnosis always paired sera about 2ml should be collected at an interval of 21 days.

d) When death is recorded, the post - mortem examinations should be conducted at the earliest to avoid putrefaction.

Points to be considered during collection of samples.

For BACTERIOLOGICAL examination/isolation: Heart blood, tissue pieces (portion of heart, livery, lung, kidney, spleen *etc.*) should be collected aseptically. Initiative should be taken to despatch the collected material as early as possible, maintaining cold chains.

For VIROLOGICAL examination/isolation: Blood, serum, tissue samples (target organ/affected site). urine, faeces, milk *etc.* may be collected aseptically during the early stage of the disease. The samples collected for virological examination may be preserved temporarily at – 20°C.For long term preservation the sample should be kept at – 80 °C. The samples collected for virological examination should be sent to the laboratory in viral transport media (PBS *etc.*) maintaining cold chains with antibiotics to check bacterial contamination.

For HISTOPATHOLOGICAL examination: Tissue samples 0.5 " to 1 " thick should be collected from the organs showing gross lesions from the margins of the lesions. After collection the samples should be sent to the laboratory in 10 per cent formalin in a wide mouth container. The tissue samples should not float. To avoid putrefaction absorbent cotton may be placed over the samples.

For TOXICOLOGICAL examination: Fresh tissue samples from kidney, liver, spleen, heart, portion of intestine, stomach content *etc.* The materials collected for Toxicological examination may be sent to the laboratory in ice or in preservative. (Rectified spirit or super saturated solution of NaCl). In that case the sample of the preservative should be sent in a separate container.

COLLECTION OF BLOOD FOR CLINICAL EXAMINATION

Type of Animal	*Veins to Select*
Cattle/Buffalo	Jugular Vein
Horse	Jugular Vein
Sheep	Jugular Vein
Goat	Jugular Vein
Pig	Ear Vein and Anterior Vena Cava
Cat	Ear vein
Dog	Cephalon Vein (Fore Limb) Recurrent Tarsal Vein (Hind Limb)

Type of Animal	*Veins to Select*
Rabbit/Guinea Pig/Mice	Ear Vein/Heart
Poultry	Wing Vein/Heart
Duck	Jugular Vein

For collection of blood the collection site should be prepared by removing hair or feather and disinfect the area with any disinfectant. Blood may be collected by sterile syringe (5/10 ml) or using vacutainer.

For serum the collected blood may be transferred in a sterile test tube and kept in a slanting position. Vacutainers containing clot activator are commonly used for separation of serum. After clotting the liquid portion is collected as serum.

COLLECTION OF MILK SAMPLES

For the diagnosis of mastitis and anti-microbial sensitivity test, milk samples collected from suspected animals BEFORE THE USE OF ANTIBIOTICS.

a) Clean the udder with soap and water
b) Wipe it with a clean cloth soaked in a disinfectant.
c) Allow to dry
d) Paint the teat orifice with Tincture Iodine or 70 per cent alcohol and allow to dry.
e) Label the sterile container with RF, RH, LF, LH
f) Discard first few stripping and collect 10 ml milk directly in the sterile container.
g) The milk sample should be sent to the laboratory immediately after collection maintaining cold chains.

COLLECTION OF FAECAL SAMPLES

Examination of faeces sample is important in case of G.I tract disorder to get information particularly about different parasites including coccidia.

Faeces should be collected in a clean container. Contamination of urine should be avoided. Samples should be collected either directly from rectum or freshly voided.

For parasitological examination samples may be sent in 10 per cent formalin and 2.5 per cent potassium dichromate solution may be used for culture of coccidial oocyst.

For Toxicological, Virological and Bacteriological examination no preservative is needed. Sample should be sent maintaining cold chains.

During collection of intestinal content two ends of a suitable portion of the intestine tide with sterile thread then cut and collected in suitable container.

COLLECTION OF SKIN SCRAPPING

The infected area of the skin disinfects first with the spirit or 70 per cent alcohol. A sterile scalpel is used to remove required tissue material and put it in the sterile container with transport medium (PBS) for virological examination. For example, goat Pox, LSD *etc.*

For Parasitological examination scrapping are taken from the affected area with the help of a scalpel or with a sharp - edge spoon. The area selected for scrapping should be at the edge of the visible lesions and their hair should be clipped away. It is useful to moisten the skin with liquid paraffin so that the scraping adheres to the scalpel. Scraping should be continued until the blood oozes from the surface.

The sample can be sent in non-absorbent paper or polythene bag. Cold chain maintain is not required for parasitological examination.

COLLECTION OF URINE

The urethra is washed and the urine is collected directly in a sterile container by CATHETOR or mid-portion of urination, The urine sample should be sent to the laboratory maintaining cold chains.

Camphor, Thymol, Formalin, Boric Acid, and Chloroform may be used as preservative in blood for routine testing.

*For BACTERIOLOGICAL AND VIROLOGICAL EXAMINATION no need of PRESERVATIVE.

COLLECTION OF PUS AND EXUDATE

Samples of sputum (Discharge from Nasal Orifices), uterine discharges should be collected with sterile cotton swab or in sterile test tube maintaining cold chains.

LYMPH NODE SMEAR

For detection of haemoprotozoal disease, examination of lymph node smear is very important. For preparation of lymph node smear, we have to locate the position of the lymph node and hold it firmly and prepare the area surgically. By means of syringe and needle pierce the gland and move the needle tip around. Pull the plunger of the syringe to aspirate the sample of the content of the gland and withdraw the needle. Expel the content to a clean slide and make the smear.

406. Describe the materials to be collected in different diseases for laboratory examination.

Answer:

MATERIALS TO BE COLLECTED FOR VIROLOGICAL EXAMINATION

Name of Diseases	*Type of Samples*
F M D	☆ Vesicular fluid in Transport Medium on ice ☆ Vesicular epithelium *i.e.* tongue, gum, dental pad lesion in 50 per cent glycerin phosphate buffer saline on ice. At least 1 gm tissue is required for diagnosis. ☆ 10 ml blood in anti- coagulant at height of temperature. ☆ Pieces of heart and other organs from calves in 10 per cent neutral formal saline solutions
LSD	☆ Blood in anticoagulant during viraemia ☆ Scabs in sterile container on ice, in 50 per cent buffered glycerin or virus transport medium ☆ Needle aspirations from skin lumps in normal saline or PBS ☆ Skin lesion in 10 per cent neutral formal saline separately ☆ Paired serum samples ☆ Post- mortem samples: Prescapular lymph node, esophagus, lung, liver, intestine, uterus *etc.* In virus transport medium and separately in 10 per cent
Rabies	☆ Half of the brain, salivary gland in 50 per cent phosphate buffered glycerin on ice in leak proof hard box and ☆ Rest half of the brain in 10 per cent neutral formal saline solution. ☆ Small pieces of hippocampus and brain (cerebellum, medulla, cerebrum, spinal cord) in 50 per cent buffered glycerin and 10 per cent neutral formal solution separately duly sealed and packed in thick poly bag and hard box labeled " Suspected for Rabies" ☆ ALL STAFF ATTENDING POST- MORTEM BE VACCINATED AGAINST RABIES.
Ephemeral Fever	Blood in EDTA on ice and paired serum sample
Cow/Buffalo Pox	☆ Scabs in sterile containers on ice ☆ Scabs in 50 per cent phosphate buffered glycerin saline and ☆ On 10 per cent neutral formal saline

Name of Diseases	*Type of Samples*
I B R (Infectious Bovine Rhinotracheitis) I P V (Infectious Pustular Vulvovaginitis)	☆ Nasal, Conjunctival and Genital swab and Foetal Tissue in transport medium ☆ Affected trachea, turbinate bones, foetal tissue in Transport Medium and in 10 per cent neutral formal saline. ☆ Paired serum samples on ice ☆ Semen and Preputial washing in Transport Medium ☆ and Paired serum on ice.
BVD	☆ Blood in E D T A ☆ Paired serum samples ☆ Semen ☆ Intestine, Lymph node and Spleen on ice ☆ Pieces of brain, liver, spleen, kidney, and nasal mucosa in 10 per cent Formalin.
Infectious Canine Hepatitis (ICH)	☆ Lung, Liver, Gallbladder, Spleen, Kidney, in PBS on ice ☆ Separately in 10 per cent formal saline.
Canine Distemper	☆ Spleen and Liver in PBS/Transport Medium on ice ☆ Pieces of Lung, Urinary Bladder, Liver, Trachea, Stomach wall and Brain in 10 per cent formal saline.
Canine Parvovirus	☆ Pieces of Liver, Spleen, Intestine, Stomach and Lymph nodes in 50 per cent Phosphate buffered glycerin saline ☆ All the stated pieces of organ in 10 per cent neutral formal saline solution.
PPR	☆ Swab from eyes, gum, rectum in PBS on ice ☆ Blood (5 ml) in anti coagulant at height of temperature ☆ Blood without anti- coagulant (5 ml) ☆ Prescapular lymph node, Spleen, pieces of Intestine on ice ☆ Lung, liver, spleen, tonsil in 10 per cent neutral formal saline solutions.
Goat Pox	☆ Skin scab with underlying tissue appears within the 1st week of clinical symptoms observed on ice ☆ Scabs in 50 per cent phosphate buffered glycerin saline ☆ Skin lesion in 10 per cent neutral formal saline solutions
Swine Fever	☆ Heparinized blood at the height of temperature in sterile container ☆ Serum on ice from live animal ☆ Spleen, lymph node, tonsil and Pancreas in 50 per cent phosphate buffered glycerin saline ☆ Pieces of brain, lung, spleen, Intestine and kidney in 10 per cent neutral formal saline solutions.

Name of Diseases	Type of Samples
African Swine Fever	☆ Blood in heparin or EDTA ☆ Spleen, tonsil, kidney, lymph node on ice ☆ Paired serum sample.
Transmissible Gastro Enteritis (T G E)	☆ Faeces, small intestine, lung and udder on ice ☆ Paired serum sample maintaining cold chains
PRRSV(Porcine Reproductive and Respiratory Syndrome Virus)	☆ Lung, Liver, Lymph node, Tonsil, Heart, Brain, Ascites fluid in ice ☆ Paired serum samples maintaining cold chains
Swine influenza	☆ Nasal swab, portion of lungs, trachea in transport medium maintaining cold chains.
Equine Influenza	☆ Nasal swabs in virus transport medium ☆ B S or HBSS (Hanks' Balanced Salt Solution) on ice ☆ Paired serum sample maintaining cold chains
Equine Infectious Anemia	☆ Blood and serum sample on ice ☆ All internal organ in 10 per cent neutral formal saline solutions
African Horse Sickness	☆ Blood in E D T A ☆ Paired serum samples maintaining cold chains ☆ Portion of spleen, brain, lung in 50 per cent phosphate buffered glycerin saline ☆ Same materials also in 10 per cent neutral formal saline solutions
Equine Encephalitis	☆ Citrate blood in ice. ☆ Paired serum samples maintaining cold chains ☆ Brain on ice

COLLECTION OF SAMPLES FOR BACTERIOLOGICAL EXAMINATION

Name of Diseases	Type of Samples
Anthrax	☆ Blood from causal vein in syringe in ice ☆ Stained and unstained bloods ear ☆ Scrapping of soil surface contaminated by the terminal discharges by the infected animal
HS	☆ Heart blood in ice ☆ Portion of liver, lung, spleen and kidney in ice ☆ Blood smear from heart blood and smear from fluid of swelling of throat, drawn by a syringe. ☆ From live animals, whole blood in glucose broth with 0.5 per cent SPS (Sodium Polyanethole Sulfonate) at febrile conditions

Name of Diseases	*Type of Samples*
BQ*	☆ Pieces of muscle from the deep of the affected muscle ☆ Tissue fluid and swab from infected muscle in transport medium specific for anaerobic. ☆ Impression smear from affected muscle.
Brucellosis	☆ Paired serum samples ☆ Vaginal mucus, seminal plasma, uterine fluid. ☆ Blood and stomach content of the aborted fetus ☆ Placenta with 3 - 4 cotyledons, vaginaly swab in PBS ☆ If possible, the whole aborted fetus on ice.
Tuberculosis	☆ Cough material from infected animals in sterile vial on ice. ☆ Milk from infected udder ☆ Faeces in sterile screw cap container ☆ Smear from lymph gland showing nodular lesion ☆ Lung, lymph gland, intestine, mesenteric lymph glands should be collected in 10 per cent formalin if lesions are observed.
Paratuberculosis (Johne's disease)	☆ Rectal pinch smear or swab ☆ Smear from thickened areas of intestine (Ileocecal valve), small portion of bowel washing (10 gm) showing gross lesions in 10 per cent formalin. ☆ Smears and pieces of mesenteric lymph nodes.
Leptospirosis	☆ Blood smear, whole blood and serum sample in ice ☆ Portions of liver, spleen and kidney showing lesion in ice and 10 per cent Formalin.
Actinomycosis	☆ Pus from mandible and maxilla in ice ☆ Smear from pus ☆ portion of mandible and maxilla showing lesion of swelling
Actinobacillosis	☆ Pus from hard swelling of tongue and lymph node
Tetanus	☆ Smear from the exudate/wound ☆ Pieces of muscle, spinal cord and brain in transport medium and in 10 per cent formalin separately.
Glanders	☆ Serum maintaining cold chains ☆ Nasal discharge in sterile swabs maintaining cold chains ☆ Portions of lungs and superficial lymph node in ☆ P B S and in 10 per cent formalin separately.

Name of Diseases	Type of Samples
Swine Erysipelas	✰ Portions of liver, lung, spleen, tonsil, lymph node heart, joint and kidney in sterile container on ice. ✰ All the stated organs in 10 per cent formalin ✰ Serum samples maintaining cold chains.
Theileriosis	✰ Smear of blood and superficial lymph nodes ✰ Smear of lymph node, spleen, liver, ✰ Portions of lymph node, spleen and abomasum in 10 per cent formalin.
Babesiosis	✰ Whole blood in ice and blood smear ✰ Smears of heart, spleen and kidney. ✰ Portions of affected visceral organ in 10 per cent formalin.

407. Describe the process how to handle the samples for Forensic Examination.

Answer: Handling samples for forensic examination involves a scientific process of elimination in investigating unnatural deaths, such as animal poisoning. Clinical findings should be present, including common symptoms such as salivation, pupil dilation, trembling, incoordination, diarrhea, hyperthermia, convulsions, paralysis, colic, abdominal pain, dry mouth, twitching, titanic spasm, labored breathing, and salivation. The intensity of poisoning and the onset of symptoms depend on the dose, mode of administration, nature of poison, age, and health of the animal.

The PM finding will clearly indicate the death of gun-shot injuries on poisoning. The sudden outbreak of symptoms followed by quick death normally indicates suspected poisoning, The autopsy of post-mortem examination is to be carried out for specific findings on the nature of poisoning or death by order means *viz.* Congestion of organs, Colour and smell of contents in stomach, nature of injuries. Bullet holes and mark of burning due to entry and exit of bullets, cyanosis oedema. P.M staining colour of blood, condition of cell membrane, ejection of blood, saliva and forth from nostrils and mouth, condition of pupils *etc.* These observations are to be recorded in P. M report.

The proper selection of autopsy materials depends on the nature of symptoms and the effects of poison on organs, nature of poison, nature of administration and time of death. The administration of poison may occur through inhalation, Ingestion, injection. Administration through mouth or rectum and through skin. In general, it occurs through ingestion.

The defense mechanism of the living system tries to counteract the effect of poison in doing so reactions are exhibited in the form of signs and symptoms. Poisons are detoxified in liver to a definite extent or eliminated though urine *i.e.*, excretory system. The elimination may also occur through saliva, stool or vomit, When the dose in above the tolerance level. The excess of poison remains absorbed in different organs *i.e.*, stomach, liver, kidney or kidneys are normally collected and preserved, these may be preserved preferably in same container (if the weight does not exceed 2 Kg.) otherwise separate containers may be used.

The nature of stomach contents of food/plant materials/remnants of tablets/ other solid materials. Their colours, smell is also good indication of suspected poisoning. The excessive secretion of saliva or ejection of stool or urine or vomit is also an important indication. The portion of skin at affected areas (preserved in saturated saline *i.e.* in case of poisoning by injection or gun-shot) in addition to blood sample (materials of chaise in case of poisoning by inhaled gases or injection). However, the other portions of viscera *i.e.*, intestine, gall bladder, Heart and lung (in case of exposure in toxic gases or poisoning by cyanogenetic glucosides)

After selection of organs (portion of animal viscera), the materials are to be collected in air- tight glass/plastic container (glass containers are preferred). Preserved, sealed (same as forwarding seal), labelled with description in details *viz*. Name and description of animal. Mark of exhibit and P. M No and date as stated in forwarding Memo, A sample of preservative is also to be sent invariably along with the above sample. The preservation may be done either by rectified spirit or super saturated saline (40 gm of common salt in 100 ml water) However rectified spirit is preferred. Formalin should never be used.

The sample thus prepared (properly sealed, labelled) are to be forwarded to F.S.L along with duly filled in and signed forwarding Memo. Detailed PM examination report and brief history of the case.

The autopsy surgeon or the concerned Head/Director/Dy. Director/ Conservator/Dy. Chief conservator/of a forest ranger/Veterinary surgeon may refer cases directly, IF THIS FALL OUTSIDE THE AMBIT OF CRIMINAL ACTS. In case of criminal poisoning exhibits are to be forwarded through the judicial Authority, In that case. The forwarding memo. Labels, certificate of authority (Empowering Director, FSI to take part of whole of exhibit/exhibits) Is required for the purpose of examination.

ANNEXURE-I

P.M EXAMINATION REPORT

Observation and points to be covered:

1. P.M no. and dated..
2. Brief history..
3. Description of viscera (portion collected) (1)(2)(3)(4)...............................
4. Name of preservative used...
5. Copy of Label and lac Seal (Specimen to be affixed)......................................
6. Mode and date of dispatch
   Information on animal. name. age. colour *etc.* ....
7. Appearance of body ....
8. Sign of decomposition...
9. Wounds and Bruises ....position, character and size..
10. State of natural orifices..
    (Eye, Ear, Nostrils, Ex. Ejection, salivation. Frothing blood. If any. Mouth. Vagina.)
11. State of limb...
12. Rigor mortis...
13. Position of
    Limbs ....
    Eyelids...
    Pupils...
    Mouth ....
    Tongue...
    Pleura ....
14. Heart: Shape and appearance...
15. Lungs, colour, consistency..
16. Position of larynx ....

17. Condition of liver. Spleen. And kidneys, intestine
(Condition of wall, Congestion, if any) ....
18. Stomach (description of colour, smell of contents to be given) ....
19. Generative organs ....
20. Condition of head ....
21. Condition of spinal cord ....
22. Fractures and dislocations ....
23. Details of injury and disease ....
24. Opinion for cause of death/health ....

Signature

Seal

ANNEXURE-II

LABEL

EXIBIT- MARKED' A

Identification of dead animal

Sex: M/F Age

P.M No. And date

Case Reference

Contents of jar : i) Stomach with contents

ii) Portion of liver

iii) Portion of kidneys

iv).

v).

Preserved in saturated saline/rectified Spirit

Signature of the Vety. Officer with rubber stamp

LABEL

EXIBIT- MARKED' B

Identification of dead animal

Sex: M/F Age

Case Reference

Sample preservative used in the viscera

Contents of jar

Preserved in saturated saline/rectified Spirit

Signature of the Vety. Officer with rubber stamp

LABEL

EXIBIT- MARKED' C

Identification of dead animal

Sex: M/F Age

P.M No. And date

Case Reference

Sample preservative used in the viscera

Contents of jar

Blood with Preserved

Signature of the Vety. Officer with rubber stamp

LABEL

EXIBIT- MARKED' D

Description of exhibit (as per forwarding Memo)

Case ref. Date.

Signature of the Vety. Officer with rubber stamp

ANNEXURE- III

FORMAT OF FORWARDING MEMO

Memo No. Date.

To

The Director
State Forensic Laboratory,
Govt. of West Bengal
37/1/2 Belgachia Road
Kolkata 700037

Sub:- Chemical Examination of Exhibit related to Unnatural death
Of.. Description..
Age..

1. Brief History of the case ....
2. Criminal case registered, if any..
3. If yes case ref. With date ....
4. P.M report enclosed ....
5. Nature of exhibits collected and preserved ....

Sl.No.	*Marked as*	*Description of Exhibit*	*Where from Collected*
1.	A	Vit Viscera of aged Colour and other description *etc.*	
2.	B	Sample of preservative used in above Viscera (Name of preservative used)	
3.	C	Sample of blood/urine	
4.	D	Food sample	
5.	E	Sample of grass	
6.	F	Sample of water	

Nature of examination

1. Whether there is suspected poison in any of the exhibit? (Marked A. B. C.)
2. Specimen Lac (metal) Seal

Signature of the Vety. Officer (rubber Stamp)

CERTIFICATE OF AUTHORITY

DIRECTOR. Forensic Science lab is authorised to take any part or whole of the exhibit for examination

Signature of the Vety. Officer

(Rubber Stamp)

GUIDELINES

N. B; Point for checking prior to forwarding of case

Documents required

1. Duly filled in and signed forwarding memo with rubber stamp impression of designation
2. Certificate of authority (duly signed by the authority)
3. I Specimen Lac seal on forwarding memo and same seal on exhibits
4. Proper marking and description of exhibits in forwarding memo and labels on exhibit

   (With signature of authority)
5. Brief history of the case
6. Detailed P.M report indication description of animal. Age. Specific finding, portion of Viscera and materials collected.

Chapter 6

General Surgery

1. **What are the different types of suture materials? Give examples.**

   Answer: the suture materials can be classified as a) Absorbable and b) Non absorbable

   a) Absorbable: Catgut, Kangaroo tendon, Collagen, Poly glycolic acid (PGA), Polyglactin (Vicryl)

   b) Non absorbable: Silk, Nylon, Cotton, Stainless steel, Polyester, Polypropylene

2. **What is catgut?**

   Answer: It was initially referred as 'Kitgut'. It is an absorbable suture material derived from submucosa of sheep intestine or serosa of cattle intestine and treated with formalin.

3. **What is Chromic Catgut?**

   Answer: When catgut is treated with chromic acid to prolong the absorption time up to 40 days and to reduce the soft tissue reaction.

4. **Which size of catgut is used for rumen suture?**

   Answer: Size 5

5. **Which size of catgut is used for muscle and other internal tissue suture?**

   Answer: Size 3 for large animals and size 1-2 for small animal.

6. **What is the absorption duration of Polyglactin (Vicryl)?**

   Answer: 45 to 90 days.

7. **Describe the different suture techniques with examples.**

   Answer: Suture patterns can be divided into two categories: interrupted sutures and continuous sutures.

   A. Interrupted sutures

   a) Simple interrupted sutures: Most frequently used skin suturing pattern.

   b) Horizontal mattress suture: When tension anticipated, this suture is superior to a simple interrupted suture. This pattern is used in skin suturing.

   c) Cross-mattress suture: This pattern is used in skin suturing when there is more tension.

   d) Vertical mattress suture: These sutures are superior to horizontal mattress sutures in terms of there ability to endure tension.

   e) Crushing suture: This particular variety of apposition suture is appropriate for gut anastomosis.

   B. Continuous sutures

   a) Simple continuous suture: Useful for the muscles, peritoneum, subcutaneous *etc.*, but typically not advised for the skin.

   b) Continuous lock suture: Because of the "locking," the sutures securely adhere the tissues.

   c) Continuous Lembert's suture: Useful for hollow visceral organs.

   d) Connell suture: An inverted suture. Alternately, the suture goes through each border of hollow intestinal organs.

   e) Cushing suture: Same as Connell suture but the thread does not penetrate the lumen.

   f) Parker-Kerr suture: Useful for suturing of stump.

   C. Tension sutures

   a) Quill suture: These vertical mattress stitches have pieces of quill or gauze attached to each edge.

   b) Far-near and Near-far suture and Far-far and Near-near suture: Applied in skin suture for obtaining more tension.

8. **What is ligation?**

   Answer: Ligation is a type of suture used to tie arteries and veins. In almost all surgical procedures, blood vessels are ligated. Large vessels should be tied off in a manner that prevents the ligature from loosening.

9. Which suture technique is applied during intestinal anastomosis?

Answer: Crushing suture

10. Where Lambert suture is indicated?

Answer: In closure of viscera

11. Which suture is applied in correction of uterine prolapse in field condition?

Answer: Per string suture may be applied during correction of uterine prolapse. But to get better result Deep Horizontal mattress suture is applied in field condition.

12. What is contusion wound?

Answer: Blunt items can cause a contusion, which damages the subcutaneous tissues without rupturing the continuity of the skin surface.

13. What is Bruise wound?

Answer: It is characterized by capillary rupture or Echymosis in the epidermis, which results in a reddish blue or pinkish coloration of the skin.

14. What is hematoma? Give examples of hematoma.

Answer: A hematoma is an abnormal cavity containing an accumulation of blood. It are frequently brought on by damage to a peripheral vein. Subcutaneous or submucosal hematomas are commonly observed.

Most commonly hematoma seen in dog is Aural hematoma at Ear flap. In cattle also in udder sometimes the hematoma is observed in mammary vein region due to rubbing with the hard surface or butting by the calf.

15. What is avulsion wound? How would you manage an avulsion wound?

Answer: When hard tissues are loosen due to some wound, called as avulsion wound like evulsion of hoof or horn.

Management: A tourniquet is placed for about 30 minutes to prevent severe bleeding. Next, a lotion with antiseptic properties is used to clean the area. Application of a bandage soaked in antiseptic lotion at the place of wound. The following day, the bandage is removed, and the wound is then dressed with an oily dressing ointment. On alternative days, this treatment is applied. A thin coating of horn tissue can be seen developing on the wound surface after a few days. Within a few months, the horny tissue is fully developed.

16. What is myiasis or maggot wound? How would you manage a maggot wound at field condition?

Answer: Fly larva infesting the worm blooded animal's flesh are termed as Maggots. "Traumatic myiasis" or "Maggot wounds" are terms used to describe the proliferation of maggots in wounds or ulcers.

Maggot wounds are of two kinds

a) Primary Maggot wound: Flies lay gees on the wound and the larvae are produced. The larvae eat the deep fresh tissue and the wound becomes larger.

b) Secondary Maggot wound: The larvae don't go to the deeper tissue and fed on the necrosed tissue of the wound.

Management

- The wound is cleaned with luke worm water to remove dirt.
- Oil turpentine or camphor oil is applied into the wound as spray.
- The maggots will come out as Oil turpentine creates lack of oxygen into the tissue.
- After removal of maggots the dead tissues should be rubbed until fresh blood comes.
- At last any antiseptic ointment should be applied over the wound topically.
- Any gram-positive sensitive antibiotic may be given parenterally for faster wound healing.
- Inj. Ivermectin is applicable to kill maggots situated in deeper tissue as per the standard dose subcutaneously

17. State the differential diagnosis among Abscess, Cyst, Hematoma, Hernia and Tumor.

Answer:

A. Abscess:

- There will be hard or soft swelling.
- Swelling may be hot and painful.
- In needle aspiration pus will come out.
- There will be a abscess point.

B. Cyst:

- Swelling is soft, fluctuating and soft in nature.
- Slowly develops than abscess.
- No pain sensation or inflammatory signs are observed.
- In needle aspiration watery material comes out.

C. Hematoma:

- Develops immediately after injury and doughy on palpation.
- No abscess point is observed and no pain sensation is there.
- In needle aspiration blood will come out.

D. Hernia:

- ☆ There will be soft swelling which is reducible in nature.
- ☆ Hernial ring is palpated at the base of hernia.

E. Tumour:

- ☆ Swelling will be hard and without pain sensation.
- ☆ There will be no abscess point in the swelling.
- ☆ In needle aspiration blood will come out.

18. Blood from nose is known as-

Answer: Epistaxis

19. Vomiting blood is referred to as-

Answer: Haematemesis

20. Blood with faeces is known as-

Answer: Melena

21. What is nosocomial infection? State the causes and control of the same.

Answer: The infection develops after admission in the hospital is known as nosocomial infection.

Common pathogens: *Chlamydia, Mycoplasma, Klebsiella, Salmonella, Clostridium, Pseudomonas, Pasteurella etc.* are the common pathogen causing nosocomial infections.

Control: Proper sanitation should be maintained before admission of any animal and isolation of infected animals should be maintained.

22. What is hydrocephalus?

Answer: A neurological condition called hydrocephalus is characterized by atypical accumulation of cerebrospinal fluid (CSF) in the brain's ventricular system. Clinical symptoms of this disease are brought on by the consequent rise in pressure on the brain.

23. What is dermoid cyst?

Answer: Dermoid cysts commonly have hair developing on them and irritate the conjunctiva and cornea. It is an embryological disorder.

24. Why fasting is ideal before anesthesia?

Answer: To avoid the chances of aspiration the stomach of animal should be fasted for at least 12 hrs before applying anesthesia.

25. Classify the anesthetics.

Answer:

a) Local anesthesia: Applied by surface application as subcutaneous injection or intradermal route.

b) Regional anesthesia: Different nerve blocks like brachial plexus block, cornual nerve block, epidural nerve block are the common regional anesthesia.

Generally, Lignocain hydrochloride 2 per cent, Procaine hydrochloride are used in local and regional anesthesia.

c) Sedation: Sedation is given before applying local or general anesthesia. Generally tran-quilizers and sedatives are applied.

d) General anesthesia: Both gaseous and intravenous anesthesia are used. Xylazine and Ketamin hydrochlorid, Propofol are used for intravenous anesthesia and Nitrous oxide, volatile fluorinated liquids are used for gaseous anesthesia.

26. Name widely used regional anesthesia method in farm animals. Name the anesthetic drug also.

Answer: Caudal Epidural anesthesia at Sacrococcygeal (S5-C1) or first coccygeal space (C1-C2).

Drug: 2 per cent Lignocain hydrochloride.

27. Name one pre anesthetic drug with dose.

Answer: Atropine sulphate. Dose: 0.04-0.06 mg/kg

28. State the dose of Xylazine in different animals.

Answer:

- ✰ Horse: 1-2 mg/kg I/m
- ✰ Cattle and buffalo: 0.1-0.2 mg/kg I/m
- ✰ Sheep and goat: 0.1-0.3 mg/kg I/m
- ✰ Pig: 2-4 mg/kg I/m
- ✰ Dog: 0.5-1 mg/kg I/m

29. Name antidotes of Xylazine.

Answer: Yohimbine

30. What are the common complications of horn found in farm animals?

Answer:

- ✰ Avulsion of horn: The horny cover separates from the bony core. Huge bleeding may take place due to this.

- ☆ Horn cancer: Squamous cell carcinoma of horn is very common in indigenous bullock. The condition is less common in cows or bulls.
- ☆ Fracture of horn: Due to sudden mechanical injury the fracture of horn may occur. Fracture generally occurs at the base of horn in oblique manner. Bleeding management is necessary in this case.

31. In which animals the Aural hematoma observed?

Answer: Dogs with pendulous ear suffers mostly from aural hematoma.

32. What is Yoke gal? State the symptoms and management.

Answer: Chronic injury of ligamentum nuchae along with yoke pressure coupled with movement causes friction and separation the layers of skin and subcutaneous tissue. As a result, inflammatory exudate is accumulated at the neck region which is termed as "Yoke gal". Generally observed in bullock.

Symptoms: Acute inflammation is observed in acute stage and fibrosis is observed in chronic stage.

Yoke abscess: Yoke abscess is the term used to describe the pus-filled cavity that forms when a yoke gall becomes infected by any pyogenic organisms.

Yoke tumor: The yoke gall growth may continue and eventually become enveloped in fibrous tissue. This is frequently referred to as a yoke tumor.

Management:

- ☆ Fomentation with magnesium sulphate can be applied in the early phases to reduce swelling.
- ☆ In the event that an abscess has formed, surgical fluid drainage is advised. Till healing takes place, the cavity should be completely flushed and disinfected with antiseptic ointment or spray. In order to prevent further contamination, systemic antimicrobial administration is advised.
- ☆ In chronic case the fibrosed tissue may be removed by applying local anaesthesia and maintaining asepsis.

33. What is capped elbow? In which animal it is very common?

Answer: The hygroma or bursitis of elbow joint is known as capped elbow. While standing up, the elbow frequently comes into contact with the hard, uneven floor. Due to repeated exposure as a defensive mechanism the synovial fluids get accumulated in the joint and this condition develops.

In horse and dog this condition is very common.

34. What is the treatment of Capped elbow?

Answer:

- ☆ Cold application is beneficial in acute stage.

- Tight bandage may be applied at the place of swelling to restrict fluid production.
- The bursa is incised and the joint fluid is drained. To minimize the production of synovial fluid the counter irritant like Tincture Iodine is given.

35. State the causes of Capped Knee.

Answer: It is very common in cattle. Unlike horses the knee comes into contact with the hard floor in case of cattle. As a result, hygroma develops at knee joint and the condition is known as capped knee. The treatment is same like capped elbow.

36. What is choking? State the causes, clinical signs of choking.

Answer: Choking also known as esophageal obstruction by any foreign object or extra luminal abnormalities. It is typically affecting cattle, buffalo, pigs, small ruminants like sheep and goats during potato harvesting season.

Causes: Obstruction of esophagus could result from unintentionally ingesting a potato, a big lemon, an apple, or a mango seed or any other solid material. Also due to any abnormal growth of tumor like substance adjacent to esophagus and development of hernia may cause choking.

Clinical signs:

- Animal will be restless and there will be profuse salivation and panting.
- The animal will refuse the feedd and water and extend the neck.
- There will be development of bloat in ruminants after a certain period.
- Animal may die due to severe dyspnoea and respiratory failure.

37. In field condition how the cases of choking can be handled?

Answer: The gas may be removed by using GTV needle in ruminants and if the chocked material is soft then may be crushed by applying pressure. Or the stomach tube or base of banana leaf may be applied to push the material towards rumen.

In severe case oesophagotomy may be performed applying local anesthesia.

38. What is hernia? Classify hernia.

Answer: An organ or tissue protruding through an unbroken skin or covered opening is referred to as a hernia. Typically, hernial ring, sac, and hernial content are required to form a hernia.

According to the location of the hernia the nomenclature is made-

a) Umbilical hernia – Common in new born calves

b) Perineal hernia – Very common in old male dogs

c) Ventral hernia – Common in cattle and horse

d) Inguinal or scrotal hernia – Common in bitches, castrated horse, stallions *etc.*

e) Pelvic hernia – Common in cattle

f) Diaphragmatic hernia – Common in dogs, cattle and buffalo.

39. What is herniorrhaphy?

Answer: When the hernial ring is reduced by suturing the ring itself, is called as herniorrhaphy.

40. What is hernioplasty?

Answer: A biomaterial is used to repair a hernia when the hernial ring is too large to suture, is called hernioplasty. Usually proline thread or mesh, stainless steel or wire mesh is used to close the hernial ring.

41. What are the organs generally herniating in diaphragmatic hernia?

Answer: Usually reticulum herniates into the thorax and sometimes omasum, abomasum, intestine, spleen, liver may herniate into thorax due to diaphragmatic hernia.

42. What is TRP or Traumatic reticuloperitonitis?

Answer: Traumatic reticuloperitonitis, which affects cattle, is a localized inflammation by perforation of the reticulum's wall that usually occurs due to ingestion of a sharp object (such as a nail or wire).

43. State the etiology and clinical findings, diagnosis and treatment of TRP.

Answer:

Etiology:

- ☆ Metallic items that are swallowed, such as nails or wire scraps, can pierce or perforate the reticulum's wall and result in traumatic reticuloperitonitis. Reticulum contractions aid the foreign object's entry into the wall.
- ☆ When the reticulum's wall is perforated, bacteria and ingesta may escape out and contaminate the peritoneal cavity. The subsequent peritonitis usually affects a small area and frequently leads to adhesions.
- ☆ Rarer occurrences include the development of a splenic, hepatic, or diffuse peritonitis that is more severe.

Clinical findings: Clinical signs include

- ☆ An abrupt drop in milk production, moderate ruminal tympany, and the sudden onset of ruminoreticular atony.
- ☆ Increased rectal temperature, ranging from moderate to severe.

- ☆ Breathing is typically shallow and rapid, and heart rate is average or only slightly elevated.
- ☆ The elbows will be abducted and stiff.
- ☆ Jugular pulsation is seen if there is development of traumatic pericarditis then brisket edema will be developed.

Diagnosis: Diagnosis is done in field condition by using a portable metal detector, Xray or USG.

Treatment: The surgical intervention – Rumenotomy is required for complete cure.

44. State the causes, sings and treatment of Atresia ani, one of the most common surgeries in field.

Answer: In newborn calves, lambs, and kids, atresia ani is seen. It is a congenital abnormality.

The disease is characterized by absence of anus, formation of a fistula between the rectum and the reproductive tract and abnormalities of the urinary tract.

Signs:

- ☆ Affected day old animals exhibit signs of unwilling to release faces.
- ☆ Sometimes females which had been taken birth with recto vaginal fistula, passes faeces through recto vaginal fistula.
- ☆ Other symptoms include weakness, straining, and abdominal discomfort as well as abdominal distension.
- ☆ Where only anus is involved, the rectum bulging will be observed subcutaneously when new born strains to defecate.

Treatment: At the location where the anus would typically be found, a circular incision of 1 to 2 cm diameter is made through the skin and subcutaneous tissue.

↓

The rectal pouch is delicately pulled caudally with a set of tissue forceps following cautious blunt dissection.

↓

The rectal pouch is cut open and the rectal mucosa is sutured to the subcutaneous tissue with four to six interrupted sutures.

45. What kinds of dislocation are common for large animals in field condition?

Answer: Dislocation of the hip, Shoulder Dislocation and Dislocation of the patella are common in large animals at field condition.

Hip dislocation:

- ☆ Most commonly found in large animals.
- ☆ Movement that is above normal range of motion as a result of falling, slipping *etc.*
- ☆ Due to both hind limbs slipping outward, the cow occasionally experiences bilateral dislocation.

Shoulder dislocation:

- ☆ The most common causes of shoulder luxation in cattle are excessive shoulder flexion and concurrent elbow flexion during jumping or sudden falls.
- ☆ Symptoms of lameness in general. Absence of weight-bearing on the injured leg. The limb is becoming shorter palpable discomfort is found.

Patellar dislocation:

- ☆ Direct force or extremely strong muscle movements can dislocate the patella.
- ☆ The patella is displaced on the inner lip of the trochlea of the tibia due to an inward luxation.
- ☆ Patella displacement on the exterior trochlear lip is referred to as an outward luxation.

46. What is Upward fixation of patella? What is the surgical intervention required for getting remedy?

Answer: Upward fixation of patella causes the medial patellar ligament of the hind limb to shrink, which causes the animal to move jerkily. It may be unilateral or bilateral. This condition causes hereditary or due to mall nutrition. In this condition the stifle and hock cannot be flexed. Lameness recovers if the animal walks for a longer time, but aggravate after a period of rest.

Treatment:

- ☆ It is claimed that injecting Lugol's iodine solution or Tincture iodide (5 to 10 ml) into the femoro-patellar joint can be helpful in many situations.
- ☆ Medial patellar desmotomy either unilateral or bilateral as per the requirement.

47. What is fracture?

Answer: Fracture is defined as any partial or complete break in the continuity of a bone due to some trauma or some pathological conditions.

48. Classify fracture.

Answer: Facture may be classified broadly into two categories and many sub categories are there,

A. ***Depending upon external contamination:***

I. Closed fracture: Here no external wound is found and no contamination takes place. It is categorized into the following types:
   a) Complete fracture – Bone is divided into two or more parts completely.
   b) Incomplete fracture – Fracture does not take place completely.

II. Open Fracture: The fractured bone comes out penetrating the surrounding tissue. Here huge chances of contamination are there. It should be always complete fracture.

B. ***Depending upon the location and direction of fracture:***

a) Transverse fracture: Fracture will be at right angle.
b) Oblique fracture: Fracture will be at an angle except right angle.
c) Spiral fracture: Fracture takes place at diagonal curve.
d) Multiple fracture: Bone broken into more than 2 pieces.
e) Avulsion fracture: When due to fracture the attachment site of muscle, tendon or ligament is detached.
f) Green stick fracture: When one side of bone is broken but the other side is intact or bent.

49. What is compound fracture?

Answer: A compound fracture is a fracture where there will be an open wound caused due to penetration of broken bone part through muscle and skin. This type of fracture is contaminated with soil or other dirty materials and animals typically get compound fractures due to any accident.

50. What are the principles of fracture repair.

Answer: The principles to repair fracture are stated as 4R.

a) Recognition: Identification of fracture site by manual intervention or radiologically.
b) Reduction: Placing of the fractured bone parts in there normal anatomical position. There are two reduction procedures
   i) Closed reduction – applying traction and
   ii) Open reduction – Good surgical practice required, bone plating, bone pinning come into this.
c) Retention: Keeping the reduced bone segments into anatomical position for a specific period and movement is completely restricted.
d) Rehabilitation: Returning to the early position as it was earlier.

51. What are the advantages and disadvantages of using plaster of paris (POP) in fracture healing or retention?

Answer:

Advantages: It is easily available and easy to prepare. It is easily can be applied over the affected limbs.

Disadvantages: It is heavy and takes more time for retention. It is suitable for the lower portions of both limbs and can't be used on humerus or femur bone fracture.

52. What are the different types of Splints are used for retention of fracture?

Answer:

a) Metal splints: Made of aluminum and can be applied to small animals.
b) Bamboo splints: Made of bamboo stick and most commonly used in field condition for large and small ruminants.
c) PVC splints: Used in pets and ruminants.
d) Thomas splints: Mostly made of aluminum and generally used for pets.

53. What is laminitis? In which animal it is seen mostly?

Answer: Laminitis (Founder) is a condition of the delicate foot laminae. It occurs more frequently in the forelimb of horses.

54. State the etiology, symptoms and treatment of laminitis.

Answer:

Etiology:

- Consuming too much grains, such as wheat and barley, or consuming feeds high in protein can all cause enterotoxaemia.
- Immediately after doing hard work, drinking cold water.
- Excessive work
- Pneumonia, metritis, and a retained placenta may cause toxicity.
- Over dose of antibiotics may kill excessive bacteria which produce endotoxins

Symptoms:

- Sudden lameness in one or both the fore limbs of horse
- Horse can't lift the body weight in this condition and withdraw feed
- The intensity of digital pulse is high and 80-120 per minute.
- Temperature may rise up to 104°F to 106°F.

Treatment:

- ☆ Target of treatment id to remove the toxins from body. Normal saline and glucose saline are used to eliminate the toxins.
- ☆ Antihistaminic and corticosteroid are given symptomatically.
- ☆ Magnesium Sulphate and Potassium Nitrate may be given orally as laxative and activated charcoal is given orally for detoxification.
- ☆ NSAID and vasodilator (Isoxsuprine) is given to reduce acute inflammation.
- ☆ Cold water and ice pack is advised at lamina to reduce inflammation.

55. What is castration? What is the ideal age of castration for different species?

Answer: Castration is a term that refers to the removal of the testicles.

Age of castration:

- ☆ Calves: 2 months of age
- ☆ Sheep and goat: 2 months of age
- ☆ Horse: 1 year old
- ☆ Pig: 1 week of age
- ☆ Cat and dog: at sexual maturity

56. Describe the methods of castration.

Answer: There are two methods of castration – a) Closed method and b) Open method

Closed method: This method involves Burdizzo emasculator for castration. No incision is made when using a closed technique. The spermatic cord is damaged, which leads to thrombus formation in the spermatic vessels. Due to lack of blood supply the testicles, undergo gradual atrophy.

Open method: The testicle and spermatic cord are made visible by incising the skin and tunica vaginalis in the open uncovered method. The spermatic cord is then severed to remove the testicle.

The tunica vaginalis is not cut in the open-covered technique. Along with their tunica vaginalis covering, the testes and spermatic cord are removed, and the testicle is removed by severing the spermatic cord as such.

57. What is spaying?

Answer: Spaying or oopherectomy refers to the removal of the ovaries.

Purpose of spaying: To restrict uncontrolled birth of puppies, to treat neoplastic or cystic changes of ovary, spaying is done in bitches.

58. What are urethral calculi?

Answer: In sheep and goat, calculi can occasionally be found at the tip of the penis, in the process urethra. The urethral process where the calculi are lodged is amputated as a treatment in these case.

59. What is the common indication of Rumenotomy?

Answer: Foreign body reticulitis or TRP, severe impaction, accidental ingestion of plastic bags, rope *etc.*

Chapter 7

Animal Nutrition

1. **Classify different animal feed ingredients with examples**

Answer:

A. Roughage (CF > 18 per cent, TDN <60 per cent):

a) Dry roughage: (Moisture content 10-15 per cent)
   i. Hay
   ii. Straw
b) Green roughage or succulent(Moisture 60-90 per cent)
   i. Pasture
   ii. Green fodder
      a) Legumes (Cowpea, cluster bean, greenpea, berseem, lucerne)
      b) Non legume (Fodder of jowar, maize, bajra, oat *etc.* and grasses of sudan, napier, guinea *etc.*)
   iii. Tree leaves
   iv. Silage
   v. Root crops

B. Concentrate (CF<18 per cent, TDN > 60 per cent)

a) Protein rich concentrate (CP >18 per cent)
   i) Animal byproducts: Blood meal, other meat scraps and offals from slaughter house, MBM, Fish meal)
   ii) Marine byproducts
   iii) Avian byproducts

iv) Brewer's grains and yeast: Dried distillers' grains and solubles

v) Oil cakes: Mustard oil cake, Ground nut cake, Soyabean *etc.*

b) Energy rich concentrate (CP<18 per cent)

i) Grains and seeds: Maize, barley, sorghum *etc.*

ii) Mill by products: Arhar chuni, wheat bran, rice bran, gram chuni *etc.*

iii) Roots: Tapioca tubers, turnip, potatoes *etc.*

Different types of Fodder Crops

1. Kharif fodder: Sorghum, Maize, Bajra,Teosinte, Sunnhemp, Cowpea
2. Rabi fodder: Oats, Lucerne, Berseem
3. Improved legumes: Berseem, Lucerne, Kudzu vine.
4. Fodder grasses: Napier, Guinea, Rhodes, Para, Anjan, Sudan
5. Fodder trees: Babul, Subabul, Sesbania, Glyricida.

2. What is gross energy of feed?

Answer: It is the amount of heat/energy given off when a particular feedstuff is completely oxidized in a bomb calorimeter containing 25-30 atmosphere of O2.

3. What is Digestible energy (DE)?

Answer: It is the part of the gross energy of feed excluding the energy lost through faeces.

4. What is Metabolizable energy (ME)?

Answer: It is the part of total energy ingested that is actually capable of transformation in the body, excluding the energy lost through faeces, urine and fermentation gasses.

5. What is Heat Increment?

Answer: It is the amount of heat produced following food consumption when the animal remains in a thermoneutral environment. It includes Heat of fermentation and heat of nutrient metabolism.

6. What is Net Energy?

Answer: It is the amount of energy that is available to the animal for maintenance and production.

NE = Metabolizable Energy- Heat increment

7. What is Biological value of Protein?

Answer: It is the percentage of nitrogen absorbed that is retained by the animal.

$$BV = \frac{\text{N intake} - (\text{Faecal N} + \text{Urinary N})}{\text{N intake} - \text{Faecal N}} \times 100$$

8. **What is NPR or Net Protein Retention?**

Answer: NPR is the ration of difference in weight loss and gain of protein non fed group and protein fed group respectively to the amount of protein consumed.

NPR = (Weight gain of protein fed group- Weight loss of Protein non fed group)/Weight of protein consumed.

9. **What is feed conversion ratio (FCR)?**

Answer: It is the amount of weight gain achieved by a particular animal per unit of food consumed. It is calculated by dividing the amount of feed consumed by the animal by its body weight gain.

10. **What is Digestible Crude Protein?**

Answer: Crude protein content is measured by multiplying N content in a feed to the factor 6.25. Digestibility coefficient is multiplied to Crude protein value to estimate Digestible crude protein.

DCP= N content* 6.25* Digestibility coefficient.

11. **Classify Carbohydrates with example**

Answer:

a) **Monosaccharides**: Monosaccharides are simple sugars. They cannot be hydrolyzed into a simpler form. The simplest carbohydrates are the three-carbon dihydroxyacetone and trioses glyceraldehyde. They are further classified into glucose, fructose, galactose, and mannose.

b) **Disaccharides**: Disaccharides are comprised of two monosaccharides connected by a glycosidic linkage (C-O-C). Cn $(H_2O)_{n-1}$ is the general formula for disaccharides. The most common disaccharides forms are lactose, sucrose, and maltose.

c) **Tri-saccharides**: Plenty of trisaccharide occur free in nature. Raffinose can be seen abundantly in many higher plants and sugar beets. Melezitose can be seen in the sap of a few coniferous trees.

d) **Polysaccharides**: Majority of the carbohydrates that can be found in nature take place as polysaccharides of high molecular weight. Polysaccharides are complex carbohydrates that are formed by the method of polymerization of a huge number of monosaccharide monomers. The other name for polysaccharides is also known as glycans.

12. How is Urea utilized by ruminants?

Answer: Urea is hydrolyzed to ammonia and carbon dioxide by the urease enzyme. Microbial fermentation of carbohydrates (primarily) yields volatile fatty acids and keto acids.

↓

Rumen bacteria use ammonia and keto acids to synthesize amino acids which are linked through peptide bonds and thus proteins are synthesized.

↓

This microbial protein is digested in abomasum and small intestine and the host animal obtains amino acids. The host ruminant builds body protein from the microbial amino acids.

↓

Optimum utilization of urea requires source of Sulphur, phosphorus, *etc.* and these factors are described hereunder.

13. What are the essential amino acids?

Answer: Essential AAs (EAAs) are synthesized by the animal itself at lower levels or not at all, and thus must be provided in the diet. For cows, the EAAs are the following: Arginine (Arg), Histidine (His), Isoleucine (Ile), Leucine (Leu), Lysine (Lys), Methionine (Met), Phenylalanine (Phe), Threonine (Thr), Tryptophan (Trp), and Valine (Val).

14. Coast disease is caused due to the deficiency of which mineral?

Answer: Cobalt

15. Which mineral is involved in propionic acid metabolism?

Answer: Cobalt

16. Which organ serves as a store house of calcium?

Answer: Bone

17. State the procedure of good quality silage preparation

Answer:

- ✰ Construct a surface/trench silo (silage storage structure). One cubic meter space/silo can store 500-600 kg of green fodder.
- ✰ Harvest the crop at 30-35 per cent dry matter (DM) stage or 65-70 per cent moisture.

- ☆ Wilt the harvested fodder to bring down DM to 30-35 per cent, if required.
- ☆ Chop the fodder into small pieces of 2-3 cm size.
- ☆ Fill the chopped fodder into the silo.
- ☆ Press the chopped fodder in the silo layer by layer of 30-45 cm.
- ☆ Filling and pressing should be completed as fast as possible.
- ☆ Use additives like molasses or urea during filling of fodder in the silo, if required.
- ☆ After filling and pressing, seal the silo with thick polyethylene sheet.
- ☆ Put weight through mud layer/sand bags/tyres on the sheet to prevent air flow beneath the sheet.
- ☆ Open the silo for feeding, minimum after 45 days, as per need.

18. **Big head disease in monkey is related to**

    Answer: Disturbance in Ca:P

19. **Nakuruitis is caused by deficiency of mineral.**

    Answer: Cobalt

20. **Chronic toxicity of selenium in cattle may cause a condition termed as**

    Answer: Alkali disease

21. **Degnala Disease is caused due to feeding of paddy straw which contains**

    Answer: Selenium

22. **Uric acid formation is impaired by the deficiency of mineral**

    Answer: Molybdenum

23. **Sheep may generally suffer from deficiency of which trace elements?**

    Answer: Copper and Cobalt

24. **Which deficiency contributes to Perosis?**

    Answer: Vitamin B12, Mn, Choline, Biotin and B10

25. **Steely and Stringy wool in sheep is due to deficiency of**

    Answer: Copper.

26. **Thumps is deficiency of Iron in which animal?**

    Answer: Piglet

27. **Falling disease is associated with chronic deficiency of**

    Answer: Copper

28. **Colostrum is an excellent source of vitamin**

    Answer: Vitamin E

29. **Nutrient deficiency leading to thumps**

    Answer: Iron

30. **Copper deficiency condition is termed as**

    Answer: Sway back/Enzootic Ataxia/Falling Disease

31. **Cereal grain byproducts generally have a higher concentration of**

    Answer: Phosphorus

32. **Which animal can tolerate massive doses of copper without showing their toxic effect?**

    Answer: Pig

33. **Which animal is most susceptible to copper toxicity?**

    Answer: Sheep

34. **Which mineral is needed to maintain the crimp in the wool?**

    Answer: Copper

35. **Selenium deficiency leads to**

    Answer: Mulberry Heart Disease, White muscle disease.

36. **ILL thrift disease is due to deficiency of which mineral ?**

    Answer: Cobalt (White liver disease)

37. **NMD in calves is deficiency of**

    Answer: Selenium

38. **All the cereal grains and their byproducts, oilseeds and oil cakes are**

    Answer: Low in Ca and High in P

39. **Grazing animals or those fed high roughage diets are more likely to be**

    Answer: Deficient in Phosphorus.

40. **Which Vitamin is involved in amino acid and carbohydrate metabolism?**

    Answer: Riboflavin

41. **Which is anti-infective Vitamin?**

    Answer: Vitamin A

42. **Nutritional Roup in poultry is deficiency of**

    Answer: Vitamin A

43. **Sulphur is required for the synthesis of**

    Answer: Biotin and Thiamin

44. **International Chick Unit is related to**

    Answer: Vitamin D

45. **International Chick Unit contains**

    Answer: 25 nanogram Vitamin D3

46. **Penguin like squat and extreme leg weakness in hens are due to a deficiency of**

    Answer: Vitamin D

47. **Soft, easily bent bones and rubbery beak in poultry are the symptoms of**

    Answer: Vitamin D deficiency

48. **Curled toe paralysis in chicks is due to deficiency of**

    Answer: Vitamin B2

49. **Internal haemorrhages due to aortic rupture in poultry is due to deficiency of**

    Answer: Vitamin K

50. **A severe oedema characterized by an increase in capillary permeability termed as 'Exudative Diathesis' in chicks is due to deficiency of**

    Answer: Vitamin E and Se

51. **Muscular Degeneration and White Muscle Disease In poultry is due to deficiency of**

    Answer: Vitamin E and Se

52. **Enlarged hock disorder (Tibiotarsal joint) in turkey is due to**

    Answer: Vitamin E and Niacin Deficiency

53. **Frizzled and rough feathers in chicks and poults is due to deficiency of**

    Answer: Calcium, Niacin and Pantothanic acid

54. **Eyelids stuck together and cheesy exudates from eyes in chicks and poults is due to**

    Answer: Vitamin A deficiency

55. Condition like Parrot Beak and chondrodystrophy in poultry's embryo is due to

Answer: Deficiency of Biotin

56. Egg White Injury preventing factor is

Answer: Biotin

57. Yeast eluating factor is

Answer: Vitamin B6

58. Anti-sterility vitamin is

Answer: Vitamin E

59. Animal protein factor name is given to

Answer: Vitamin B12

60. Vitamin C is dietary essential in

Answer: Human, monkey and Guneapig

61. Mulbery heart disease in pig is caused due to deficiency of

Answer: Vitamin E

62. Chicken sits on its flexed legs and draws its head backward (Star grazer) is due to

Answer: Deficiency of Thiamin

63. Polioencephalomalacia and cerebro cortical necrosis in ruminants are caused by

Answer: Deficiency of Thiamin.

64. Pelegra or blue lounge in man is caused due to deficiency of

Answer: Niacin

65. Black tongue in dog is due to

Answer: Niacin deficiency

66. Clubbed down condition in chicken embryo is due to

Answer: Riboflavin deficiency

67. Goose stepping in pig is due to deficiency of

Answer:Pantothanic acid

68. Which species is unable to convert beta carotene to vitamin A

Answer: Cat

69. Bitot Spot is seen due to deficiency of

Answer: Vitamin A

70. Stiff Lamb disease is related to deficiency of

Answer: Vitamin E and Se

71. Yellow fat disease in cat is due to deficiency of

Answer: Vitamin E

72. Chastek paralysis is caused due to deficiency of

Answer: Vitamin B1

73. Fatty liver and kidney syndrome in chicken is caused by deficiency of

Answer: Biotin

74. Crooked calf disease is caused by the ingestion of

Answer: Quinolizidine.

75. Liver damage can be assessed by the activities of

Answer: AST and ALT

76. First limiting Amino acid in pig diets is

Answer: Lysine.

77. The straws are poorly digestible because they contain high amount of

Answer: Lignin.

78. Feeding of excess lipids/oils in the ration of ruminants affect the digestibility

Answer: Fiber.

79. Posterior Paralysis in pig is due to deficiency of

Answer: Phosphorus and Calcium

80. Mention the NRC specifications of various nutrients for poultry.

Nutrients	*Broiler Starter (0-4wks)*	*Broiler Finisher (4-8wks)*	*Pullet (0-6 wks)*	*Pullet (6-14 wks)*	*Pullet (14-20 wks)*	*Layer/ Breeding Hens*
ME (kcal/kg)	3200	3200	2900	2900	2900	2850
CP per cent	23	20	20	16	12	15
Calorie/ protein ratio	139:1	160:1	137:1	158:1	190:1	190:1
Calcium per cent	1.0	1.0	0.8	0.8	0.8	Layer -2.75 Breeder-0.75

81. What is the optimum Linoleic acid percentage for maximum egg size?

Answer: 1 per cent of linoleic acid in the diet.

82. Which is essential for prevention of perosis in Chicken?

Answer: Choline.

83. Which amino acid is essential only in birds?

Answer: Glycine

84. Feather protein contains high amount of

Answer: Cystine

85. Mention different vitamin deficiency symptoms in Poultry.

Sl.No.	*Nutrients*	*Deficiency symptoms*
1	Thiamin (Vitamin B1)	Polyneuritis (star grazing), Chastek paralysis
2	Riboflavin (Vitamin B2)	Curled toe paralysis
3	Niacin (Vitamin B3) and Pyridoxine (Vitamin B6)	Chondrodystrophy
4	Vitamin B12	Gizzard erosion
5	Vitamin A	Night blindness, Xerophthalmia
6	Vitamin K	Impaired clotting system
7	Folic Acid	Loss of feather pigmentation
8	Biotin	Dermatitis-severe lesions on bottom of feet in early stages and mandibular lesion at later stage.
9	Pantothanic Acid	Dermatitis-mandibular lesion at early stages and mild lesions at feet at a later stage.
10	Vitamin E	Crazy chick disease, encephalomalacia, Exudative diathesis
11	Vitamin D	Rickets in young chicken, Osteomalacia in adult bird
12	Niacin or Zinc	Slipping of gatrocnemius or achilies tendon from condyles, Hock enlargement.
13	Niacin	Bowed leg in Duck
14	Vitamin D	Penguin like squat
15	Folacin	Macrocytic Hyperchomicanaemia
16	Vitamin K deficiency	Internal haemorrhage from aortic rupture.

86. What is the function of glycin in birds?

Answer: Biosynthesis of uric acid

87. What are the two semi essential amino acids in Birds?

Answer: Cysteine (can be obtained from Methionine) and Tyrosine (Can be obtained from Phenylealanine)

88. What is the function of arginine in poultry?

Answer: Arginine is essential in poultry and yields urea and ornithine on metabolism.

89. Which factors determine the size of egg?

Answer: Level of dietary protein and linoleic acids

90. Mention different Mineral deficiency symptoms in poultry

Sl.No.	*Mineral*	*Symptoms*
1.	Zn	Frizzled and rough feather
2.	Se	Exudative Diathesis
3.	Na	Cannibalism
4.	I	Enlarged Thyroid
5.	Mn	Reduced egg shell strength
6.	P	Cage layer fatigue
7.	Mg	Hyperirritability
8.	Chloride	Characteristic fright reaction with titanic spasm.
9.	Cu	Enlarged heart
10.	Zn or Mn	Shortening and thickening of leg bones in chicks
11.	Mn, Choline, Folacin, Biotin, vitamin B12, or Zn	Perosis or slipped tendon in chicks
12.	Fe/Cu	Microcytic, Hypochromic, anemia

91. Which water soluble vitamin is stored in the chicken body?

Answer: Vitamin B7

92. For prothrombin production which vitamin is needed?

Answer: Vitamin K

93. Which is a Vitamin K antagonist leading to hemorrhagic spots or bleeding?

Answer: Sulfa drugs

94. Bowing of the legs with an enlarged hock joint without slipping of the Achilles tendon is due to

Answer: Choline deficiency.

95. Which is needed for maturation of RBC in poultry?

Answer: Folic acid

96. Rough and scaly dermatitis on the bottom of the chick foot is due to deficiency of

Answer: Biotin.

97. Which vitamin is needed as supplementation only in summer stress for poultry?

Answer: Ascorbic acid.

98. Cage layer fatigue is severe with

Answer: Low calcium and excess phosphorus.

99. Mention the level of inclusion of feed sources in poultry diets.

Sl.No.	*Feed Ingredients*	*Chicks and Broiler*	*Grower and Layer*	*Remarks*
1.	Soyabean Meal	35	25	Can be used as the sole source of protein
2.	Peanut meal	35	25	Prone to contaminate with mycotoxins
3.	Cotton Seed Meal	10	10	Iron supplementation is required to bind Gossypol
5.	Coconut meal	03	05	Prone to mycotoxin contamination
6.	Rape seed/Mustered meal	03	05	Erucic acid, Tannins, glycosylates are present
7.	Sunflower meal	05	10	High in fiber
8.	Sesame/Til cake	10	15	High in Phytates and oxalates
9.	Linseed meal	3	5	Linatin, linamarin and indigestible mucilage
10.	Karanja cake extract	5	10	Contains Karanjin.Only solvent cakes should be used
11.	Fish meal	10	10	Rancidity, fire accidents and pathogenic microbial contamination
12.	Meat meal	5	5	Pathogenic microbial contamination
13.	Meat cum bone meal	5	5	Pathogenic microbial bone meal contamination
14.	Ground Nut Cake	5	10	Low in lysine, methionine and Tryptophan, poorly digestible.

100. The mineral that partially spares the vitamin E

Answer: Selenium.

101. Necrotic dermatitis of the chicken feet is caused by the deficiency of

Answer: Zn

102. Gossypol of Cotton Seed Meal react with

Answer: Iron

103. The major end product of nitrogen metabolism in poultry is

Answer: Uric acid

104. The major end product of nitrogen metabolism in mammals is

Answer: Urea

105. Water intake in poultry is reduced due to the deficiency of

Answer: Na

106. What is the water percentage in different feed ingredients?

Answer:

Sl.No.	*Ingredients*	*Water Percentage*
1.	Hay	12-14 per cent
2.	Straws	10 per cent
3.	Silage	60-70 per cent

107. What is the optimum water consumption and DMI: Water ratio in animals?

Answer:

Sl.No.	*Species*	*Water Intake (per day)*	*DMI : Water Consumption*
1.	Adult Cattle	30L	1:3 to 3:5
2.	Sheep and Goat	4-6 L	1:4
3.	Swine	6-8 L	1:3
4.	Poultry	250ml	1:2

108. How much water is required per litre of milk production in dairy cow?

Answer: 3 ltr

109. Excess grain feeding to ruminants results in

Answer: Ruminal acidosis

110. Name a fermentation stimulant ingredient

Answer: Molasses

111. Legumes are rich in

Answer: Calcium

112. What is Haylage?

Answer: Haylage is a high dry matter silage which is made from grass and/or legume containing a moisture level of about 45-55 per cent having a pleasant aroma, good palatability

113. Describe the chareacteristics features of Hay, Silage and Straw.

Answer:

Features	*Hay*	*Silage*	*Straw*
Moisture per cent	12-14 per cent	60-70 per cent	10 per cent
Suitable crop	Hollow stem crop which is rich in protein like Lucerne, berseem, cowpea *etc.*	Carbohydrate rich crop like maize, bajra, jowar	By product of any crop after threshing
Nature of the product	Dried	Fermented	Dried

114. Cereal grains are rich in

Answer: Phosphorus (Low in Calcium)

115. Which Vitamin can't be synthesized by Plants?

Answer: Vitamin B12

116. Where in ruminants Vitamin C, Vitamin B complex and Vitamin K are synthesized?

Answer: Vitamin C- Tissue

Vitamin B Complex- Rumen

Vitamin K- Rumen

117. Where vitamins are not all synthesized?

Answer: Monogastric animals.

118. The additives most commonly used in silage is

Answer: Molasses and Salt

119. What is DM content of Hay?

Answer: 80-85 per cent

120. What is DM content of Haylage?

Answer: 40-45 per cent

121. Which vitamin mainly lasts during Hay making?

Answer: Vitamin A

122. Suitable crop for silage making is

Answer: Zea mays

123. A good quality silage should higher proportion of

Answer: Lactic acid.

124. Thick stem crop is more suitable for making

Answer: Silage

125. Thin stem crop is more suitable for making

Answer: Hay

126. Hay should not be fed to

Answer: Pig

127. Which type of bacteria is desirable while silage making?

Answer: Lactobacilli

128. What is the minimum time required for silage making?

Answer: 1.5-2 months.

129. Paddy straw is rich in

Answer: Oxalate and Lignin

130. What is the safe inclusion level of Molasses in ruminant ration?

Answer: 5-10 per cent

131. Which crop is responsible for HCN toxicity in ruminants?

Answer: Immature Jowar

132. Nitrate toxicity is more serious in

Answer: Ruminants.

133. A term 'BRIX' commonly used to indicate

Answer: Sugar content in Molasses.

134. Honey Comb like interior structure is present in

Answer: Reticulum

135. Rumen microbes converts feed carbohydrates to VFA which are mainly absorbed from

Answer: Rumen

136. Total VFA production in rumen can be up to

Answer: 4kg/day

137. The average rate of gas production in the rumen is

Answer: 30L per hour

138. What is the percentage of Methane in rumen gases?

Answer: 25 per cent

139. A low milk fat results when the ratio of acetic to propionic acid in the rumen content falls bellow

Answer: 3:1

140. Rate of methane production in rumen for every 100 g of carbohydrate digested

Answer: 4.5g

141. What are the main toxic factors associated with feedstuffs?

Answer:

Feedstuff	*Toxic factor*
Raw Soyabean and its meal	Trypsin inhibitor, phytohaemaglutinin, antigens, lipoxigenase, goiterogen, saponin, estrogen, phytic acid and oligosaccharides (NSPs -30.3 per cent)
Groundnut and its meal	Trypsin inhibitor, Goiterogen, Tannins, oligosaccharides and lectins
Linseed and its cakes	Linamarin (cyanogenicglucoside), antipyridoxin (Linatin) and Mucilage (HCN level 10-300mg)
Cotton Seed and its meal	Gossypol cycloproenoid fatty acid
Neem seed and its meal	Limonoids, Azadirone, Nimbin, Azadirachtin
Mahua Cake	Mowrin (Saponin) and Tannins
Wheat	Tyramine, Trypsin Inhibitors, NSPs (11.4 per cent)
Rice	Estrogen and Haemaglutinins

142. Which toxic factor is present in subabool?

Answer: Mimosin.

143. Which feed has antivitamin E activity?

Answer: Kidney bean

144. Which feed has antivitamin K activity?

Answer: Sweet clover

145. Which feed has antivitamin B6 activity?

Answer: Linseed meal.

146. How much water is required for one kg of milk production?

Answer: 3-4kg

147. A high calcium intake in the diet can lead to deficiency of

Answer: Zn

148. Wool is rich in which amino acid?

Answer: Cysteine (contains 4 per cent Sulphur)

149. What is the percentage of caseins in total milk protein?

Answer: 80 per cent

150. What is the reason that caseins cannot be denatured by heating of milk?

Answer: Because casein doesn't have an organized structure.

151. What are the minerals deficient in milk?

Answer: Mg, Fe and Cu

152. Which supplementation decreases the risk of Ketosis?

Answer: Niacin supplementation.

153. What is the recommended dosage of Niacin.

Answer: 6gm of niacin per day should be fed during the last 21 days before calving and for 3 months after calving.

154. How much crude protein is required for one kg milk production?

Answer: 70gm of crude protein per kg of milk production.

155. Panting under heat stress leads to

Answer: Respiratory alkalosis

156. A high molasses diet prior to calving predisposes the animal to

Answer: Milk fever

157. Cannibalism among poultry birds occurs as a result of

Answer: Salt deficiency, amino acids deficiency, excessive light, low number of feeders *etc.*

158. Pinning condition occurs due to deficiency of

Answer: Cobalt

159. Salt lick disease develops due to deficiency of

Answer: Copper

160. Big neck disease occurs due to deficiency of

Answer: Iodine

161. Teartness condition occurs due to

Answer: Excess of Molybdenum

162. Excess feeding of Paddy straw can lead upto

Answer: Ca deficiency.

163. Parakeratosis occurs due to deficiency of

Answer: Zn

164. Lechsucht disease occurs due to deficiency of

Answer: Copper

165. The peg leg condition in grazing cattle is due to the deficiency of

Answer: Ca deficiency

166. Super juice is used in some countries as a source of

Answer: Phosphorus.

167. Deficiency of phosphorus in animals can lead to

Answer: Pica, Sarcophagia, rupturing of Achillus tendons, haemoglobinurea.

168. Big head disease is caused due to

Answer: Phosphorus excess.

169. Excess phosphorus feeding along with low calcium feeding in horse can lead to

Answer: Big head disease, Brain disease, Nutritional secondary hyperparathyroidism.

170. Which animal is more susceptible to cobalt deficiency?

Answer: Sheep.

171. Cobalt deficiency can cause

Answer: Bush sickness, Salt sick, Coast disease, Pinning disease

172. White liver disease and Phalaris staggers disease occur due to

Answer: Cobalt deficiency

173. Which mineral is highly present in lush green pasture which and when fed to animal lead to hypomagnesemia?

Answer: Potassium.

174. Nutritional chondrodystrophy in chicks occurs due to deficiency of

Answer: Manganese

175. Plumbism is toxicity of

Answer: Lead

176. Hydragyria is the toxicity of

Answer: Mercury

177. Degcure mixture used for the treatment of degnella disease is a

Answer: A penta sulphate mineral mixture.

178. Bunny Hopping, Pacing Gait, and Pigeon-Toed condition in ruminants occur due to deficiency of

Answer: Cu

179. Which vitamin is known as antirachitic vitamin?

Answer: Vitamin D

180. Polyneuritis in birds occur due to deficiency of

Answer: Thiamine

181. Vitamin H is synonymous for

Answer: Biotin

182. Which Vitamin is synthesized in poultry?

Answer: Vitamin C

183. Continuous feeding of boiled polished rice to chick may lead to

Answer: Vitamin B1 deficiency

184. Excessive feeding of Amprolium salt in poultry can results in

Answer: Vitamin B1 deficiency

185. Which poultry birds have highest requirement of Niacin?

Answer: Duck

186. Pellagra occurs in human due to deficiency of

Answer: Niacin.

187. Biotin is also known as

Answer: Vitamin B7

188. Continuous feeding of raw eggs can lead to deficiency of

Answer: Biotin

189. Egg white injury occurs due to deficiency of

Answer: Biotin.

190. Biotin antagonist present in raw egg is

Answer: Avidin

191. Folic acid is known as

Answer: Vitamin M/Factor U/Vitamin B9

192. Lactobacillus casei factor **is now known as**

Answer: Folic acid

193. Which animal is more susceptible for folic acid deficiency?

Answer: Poultry birds.

194. Which vitamin deficiency cause Megaloblastic anaemia?

Answer: Folic acid and Vitamin B12

195. For human which deficiency is most common?

Answer: Vitamin B9 or Folic acid deficiency

196. Vitamin B12 is also known as

Answer: Cyanocobalamin, Animal Protein Factor and Chick growth factor.

197. Which Vitamin is Known as 'Lipotrophic factor'

Answer: Choline

198. Which Vitamin prevents fatty liver formation?

Answer: Choline

199. Spraddled leg condition in swine can occur due to deficiency of

Answer: Choline.

200. Which vitamin is involved in the synthesis of collagen?

Answer: Vitamin C

201. Xeropthalmia occurs as a result of a deficiency in

Answer: Vitamin A

202. Which animal is more efficient in conversion of carotene to Vitamin A?

Answer: Poultry Birds

203. Which vitamin is known as " anti-infective " Vitamin?

Answer: Vitamin A

204. "Pink eye condition " in ruminants occur due to deficiency of

Answer: Vitamin A

205. Nyctalopia condition can occur due to deficiency of

Answer: Vitamin A

206. Rachitic Rosary condition occur due to deficiency of

Answer: Vitamin D

207. Yellow fat disease (steatitis) occurs due to deficiency of

Answer: Vitamin E

208. Bleeding disease occur due to deficiency of

Answer: Vitamin K

209. Cheilosis in human occur due to deficiency of

Answer: Riboflavin

210. Braken Fern poisoning in horse cause the deficiency of which Vitamin?

Answer: Thiamine.

211. Xerosis occur due to deficiency of

Answer: Vitamin A

212. Corn bred fever occur due to deficiency of

Answer: Niacin

213. Excess intake of Molybdenum results in which mineral deficiency?

Answer: Copper

214. Which mineral is abundant in legumes but deficient in cereals?

Answer: Calcium

215. Which pigment of Maize is responsible for yellow colour of egg yolk?

Answer: Zeaxanthin

216. Which vitamin deficiency may result in early embryonic mortality?

Answer: Thiamin

217. Calcium content in layer ration is

Answer: 3 per cent and above

218. Colour of Good Silage is

Answer: Yellowish or brownish green.

219. Silo-filter's disease is an illness to farmers due to inhalation of

Answer: Oxides to Nitrogen.

220. Legume hay differs from non-legume hay as it contains

Answer: High protein and high Calcium

221. Cereal grains are deficient in which amino acid?

Answer: Lysine

222. Which vitamin is mainly lost during hay production?

Answer: Vitamin A

223. When steaming up is practiced?

Answer: It is practiced 2 months before expected lambing (Start with 100gm increase 100 gm every 15 days till lambing).

224. What are the standards of organic livestock production?

Answer:

a) Breeding management: Local breeds are preferred. Natural mating is preferred although AI is also permitted.

b) Housing management: Loose housing system is preferred.

c) Health Management: Herbal, homeopathic or ayurvedic products are preferred over allopathic medicine. Mutilation such as tail docking, cutting of teeth, trimming of beaks *etc.* are not permitted. However, disbudding, castration, hoof trimming, cutting of needle teeth in pigs *etc.* are permitted.

225. How far cattle can be driven by foot?

Answer: 30-35 km per day.

226. What is Bagging?

Answer: Bagging is leaving milk in the udder for 6 or more hours to keep the udder in shape before show and judging.

227. What is challenge feeding?

Answer: It is the feeding of high yielders cattle, two weeks prior to expected date of calving with increasing quantity of concentrate mixture to challenge against negative energy and protein in the coming lactation. In order to prepare her digestive tract for the increased amount of concentrate in early lactation and provide enough nutrients to initiate lactation on higher plane. Increases of 300-400 gm of concentrate mixture every day, which is maximum upto 0.5 to 1 kg of concentrate per 100 kg of body weight, is practiced in the challenge feeding.

228. What is Defaunation?

Answer: It is the act of removing ciliate protozoa from the rumen.

229. What is Flushing?

Answer: Feeding of extra concentrate and high plane of nutrition two weeks prior to breeding season for getting multiple births in pig and sheep.

230. What is Garget milk?

Answer: Milk drawn from an animal suffering from mastitis.

231. What is Gritty or Sandy Milk?

Answer: Milk containing a high concentration of granular Ca and Mg.

232. What is Steaming Up?

Answer: Feeding of extra concentrate to the heifer or pregnant cow prior to calving.

233. What is Zero-hour grazing?

Answer: Grazing of animals at night to avoid heat stress during the summer.

234. What is the thumb rule for urea feeding?

Answer: The amount of supplemented urea should not exceed

a) 1 per cent of total ration

b) 3 per cent of concentrate mixture

c) 33 per cent or $1/3^{rd}$ of crude protein equivalent

235. Which level of ammonia is toxic?

Answer: In blood 1mg/100ml, in rumen 80 mg/100 ml

236. How much Starch is required for urea feeding?

Answer: 1kg starch per 100 gm urea

237. What is the composition of Urea Molasses Mineral Block?

Answer: Wheat bran 40 per cent, Molasses 38 per cent, Urea 10 per cent, Binder 10 per cent, Salt and Mineral 2 per cent

238. What amounts of DCP and TDN are required for a cow weighing 400 kg and producing 10 liters of milk (4 per cent FCM) per day?

Answer:

a) For maintenance 254 gm DCP and 3.03kg TDN
b) For milk production 480gm DCP and 3.39 kg TDN
c) Total 734 gm DCP and 6.42 kg TDN

239. Determination of quality of silage

Silage Category	*pH*	*Ammonical Nitrogen*	*Lactic Acid*	*Butyric Acid*	*Acetic Acid*	*Colour*	*Odour*	*Fungus/ Moulds*
Very Good	3.5-4.2	<10 per cent	8-12 per cent of DM	NIL	0.7-4 per cent	Yellowish green	Acidic	No
Good	4.2-4.5	10-15 per cent	Less	0.2 per cent		Green or Brownish	Acidic	May/ May not
Fair Silage	4.5-4.8	15-20 per cent	Very less	0.3-0.5 per cent		Tobacco brown to dark brown	Foul	Present
Poor Silage	>4.8	>20 per cent	Least	>0.5 per cent		Blackish	Foul	Present

240. Which grass is known as elephant grass?

Answer: Pennisetum purpureum or Hybrid Napier

241. Name the ideal crop for silage making?

Answer: Maize

242. Which vitamin cannot be synthesized and is therefore essential in the diet

Answer: Vitamin E

243. The colour of cow milk is yellowish due to presence of

Answer: Carotene

244. Giving an anticoccidial drug to a calf results in deficiency of

Answer: Thiamin

245. The major VFA produced in rumen of buffalo is

Answer: Acetic acid

246. Which animal has largest caecum?

Answer: Horse

247. Enzootic ataxia is caused by the deficiency of

Answer: Copper

248. Sway back is caused by the deficiency of which nutrient?

Answer: Copper

249. Polyuria occurs due to intoxication of which vitamin?

Answer: Vit-D

250. Which vitamin deficiency causes urolithiasis?

Answer: Vit-A

251. Which vitamin helps in the absorption of iron?

Answer: Vit-C

252. Which amino acid is the most limiting for milk protein synthesis'?

Answer: Methionine

253. Pyruvate is accumulated by the dietary deficiency of which vitamin?

Answer: Vitamin B1

254. White muscle disease in calves is caused by deficiency of which vitamin?

Answer: Vit E

255. Which vitamin is most essential for utilization of propionic acid?

Answer: Vit B12

256. Falling disease occur in cattle due to deficiency of which mineral

Answer: Copper

257. Steely wool in sheep results from deficiency of which mineral or nutrient?

Answer: Copper

258. Which vitamin is dietary essential for all species?

Answer: Vit A

259. Which vitamin deficiency is associated with Bitot spopt?

Answer: Vit A

260. High amount of Rice straw feeding in high yielding pregnant cattle or lactating cattle may lead to Milk fever due to what reason?

Answer: As the oxalates present in straw affect the absorption calcium. Oxalates can be reduced after soaking straw in water before feeding.

261. What is the ratio of VFA?

Answer: Acetic acid: Propionic acid: Butyric acid=65:25:15

262. Which VFA is important for fat synthesis in milk?

Answer: Acetic acid

263. Which VFA is important for production of milk?

Answer: Propionic acid

264. What type of feed in cattle increases milk fat percentage?

Answer: More roughage feeding increase fat percentage due to more Acetic acid and VFA production.

265. Peat scours or teart in cattle occur due to which element?

Answer: Molybdenum toxicity

266. Crippling disease or Slipped tendon occur in chicks due to deficiency of which mineral?

Answer: Manganese

267. Which trace element can be found in insulin?

Answer: Zn

268. Which Vitamin deficiency is responsible for Stiff lamb disease?

Answer: Vit E

269. What is Bypass protein? Why is bypass protein more essential for high yielding animal?

Answer: The fraction of dietary protein that escapes bacterial degradation in the rumen is called Bypass protein. Degradable fraction of protein is utilized by rumen microbes for their own protein synthesis and ruminant digest these microbes for their own protein. So in case of degradable protein some fraction of protein is utilized by animal which is not sufficient for high yielding cattle. Bypass protein escapes rumen degradation and is directly utilized by animal for their own protein. So, for high yielding animal Bypass protein is more essential.

270. Alkali disease is caused by toxicity of which mineral?

Answer: Selenium

271. Crazy chick disease or Encephalomalacia occur in fowl due to deficiency of what? Why the name is Crazy Chick?

Answer: Vit E deficiency. As the diseased chick appears to push its head beneath its breast.

272. How much feed is required on a daily basis for deshi and cross bred cattle?

Answer: Though the requirement of feed/nutrients depends upon the size, stage of growth of the animal, production and other factors but a thumb rule as given below may be followed.

	Maintenance	*Lactation*
Indigenous	Concentrate. 1.5-1.75 kg with Straw 4k, 8 kg green roughage	Extra 400 gm concentrate per litre milk production
Crossbred	Concentrate. 2-2.5 kg with Straw 6 kg, Green Roughage 10-12 kg	Extra 500 gm concentrate per litre milk production

273. Give example of some leguminous and non-leguminous fodder?

Answer:

Leguminous fodder: Lucerne, Berseem

Non-Leguminous fodder: Maize, Jowar, Napier

274. What is the principal acid in silage?

Answer: Lactic acid

275. What is Azolla and what is the protein content of Azolla. How is Azolla produced for animal feeding at farmer's house?

Answer: Azolla is *an aquatic fern belonging to the plant family Azollacea* which is grown primarily as a fodder for livestock.

The protein content of azolla is 25 per cent on a DM basis.

Process for Azola cultivation:

☆ A water body is made, preferably under the shade of a tree, with the help of a plastic sheet. A pit of 2 x 2 x 0.2 m is dug as a first step.

↓

☆ All corners of the pit should be at the same level so that a uniform water level can be maintained. The pit is covered with plastic gunnies to prevent the roots of the nearby trees piercing the plastic sheet, which is spread over the plastic gunnies.

↓

☆ About 10 – 15 kg of sieved fertile soil is uniformly spread over the plastic sheet. Slurry made of 2 kg cow dung and 30 g of Super Phosphate mixed in 10 litres of water, is poured onto the sheet. More water is poured on to raise the water level to about 10 cm.

↓

☆ About 0.5 – 1 kg of fresh and pure culture of azolla is placed in the water. This will grow rapidly and fill the pit within 10 – 15 days. From then on, 500 – 600 g of azolla can be harvested daily. A mixture of 20 g of Super Phosphate and about 1 kg of cow dung should be added once every 5 days in order to maintain rapid multiplication of the azolla and to maintain the daily yield of 500g.

↓

☆ A micronutrient mix containing magnesium, iron, copper, sulphur can also be added at weekly intervals to enhance the mineral content of Azolla.

276. What is the proportion of urea molasses are used for treatment of straw?

Answer: 4kg urea+10kg molasses+40kg water for 100 kg chopped straw

277. What is Probiotic and Prebiotic

Answer: Probiotic: Probiotic is a mixed culture of living organism which helps the animal by improving the properties of its natural intestinal microflora.

Prebiotic: A prebiotic is an indigestible carbohydrate that selectively stimulates the growth or activity of one or a limited number of bacterial species already present in intestine. *e.g.* Fructo-oligosaccharide and Mannan-Oligosaccharide.

278. What is Hydroponic fodder cultivation?

Answer: Hydroponic fodder is a method used to cultivate highly nutritious sprouted grains as livestock feed using a hydroponic system instead of soil. It is straightforward way of providing all nutrients, water, sunlight without the need of soil under controlled environment condition to optimize the growth of plants. (Use mineral nutrient solution in a water solvent, roots exposed in the nutritious liquid or physically supported by an intermedium such as perlite or gravel)

Advantages:

- ☆ High nutritional value. Hydroponic fodder has high protein content and low anti-nutritional factors, making it an excellent source of feed for livestock.
- ☆ Hydroponic fodder is sustainable farming practice that requires less water and land compared to traditional crop farming.
- ☆ Less labour requirement
- ☆ Reduction in growth time of green fodder: To obtain nutritious fodder requires just over seven days from seed germination to fully grown plant 25-30cm height
- ☆ The high quality nutrients in hydroponic fodder can enhance the health and well being of livestock.
- ☆ Hydroponic fodder is a cost effective alternative to traditional feed sources.

279. What causes the difference in colour between cow milk which appears yellowish creamy white in colour and buffalo milk, which appears creamy white in colour?

Answer: Because in buffalo beta carotene pigment gets converted to colourless vitamin A, so buffalo milk is creamy white, whereas in cows, this conversion is very less, so cow milk is yellowish.

280. Which protein is responsible for the whitish colour of the milk in general?

Answer: Casein protein

281. Which immunoglobin is the most abundant in colostrum?

Answer: IgG

282. Which rumen microorganism is referred to as biological knife?

Answer: Fungi

Chapter 8

Veterinary Microbiology and Immunology

1. **Immunoglobulin associated with parasitic immunity**
   Answer: IgE
2. **The largest immunoglobulin is**
   Answer: IgM
3. **Main immunoglobulin protecting mucosal surface**
   Answer: IgA
4. **Cell mediated immunity and humoral immunity is carried out by**
   Answer: T cells and B cells, respectively
5. **Which immunoglobulin first appears in primary immune response?**
   Answer: IgM
6. **The toxic granules of Dohle's body are present in**
   Answer: Macrophage
7. **The antibody class that can pass through placenta**
   Answer: IgG 2a
8. **The antibody class that is rich in cow milk**
   Answer: IgE

9. **The temperature and duration of sterilization in a hot air oven are**

   Answer: 160°C and 1 hour

10. **The commonly used medium for the growth of fungi is**

    Answer: Sabouraud's dextrose agar

11. **A positive TB skin test denotes**

    Answer: Delayed hypersensitivity

12. **A serum containing specific antibodies in large quantity that is used in detecting antigens is**

    Answer: Hyperimmune serum

13. **Blood serum can be sterilized by**

    Answer: Filtration

14. **Agents that cause summer mastitis**

    Answer: *Streptococcus dysgalactiae* and *Corynebacterium pyogens*

15. **Kennel cough in dogs is caused by**

    Answer: *Bordotella bronchoseptica*

16. **Bioterrorism of a country is associated with**

    Answer: Anthrax

17. **Chinese letter arrangement and metachromatin granules are features of**

    Answer: *Corynebacterium diptheriae*

18. **Which organism causes abortion with necrotic placentitis and leathery placenta in cattle?**

    Answer: *Brucella abortus*

19. **Strain 19 (living) and Strain 45/20 (killed) respectively types of vaccines used against calves and cows**

    Answer: Brucellosis

20. **Bacillus antharcis has a medusa head like appearance in**

    Answer: Nutrient agar

21. **Abortion storms in sheep is caused by**

    Answer: *Campylobacter foetus*

22. **Antibiotic which can also function as an anthelmentic agent**

    Answer: Hygromycin B

23. **The commonly used agent for 'cold sterilization' is**

    Answer: Gamma radiation

24. **Dick's test employed in the detection of**

    Answer: *Staphylococcus pyogenes*

25. **9R is a vaccine strain of**

    Answer: *Salmonella gallinarum*

26. **Which is the chief source of leptospira ?**

    Answer: Urine

27. **The bacterial disease that randomly destroys a poultry farm**

    Answer: Collibacillosis

28. **Which bacterium is predisposed by** *Fasciola hepatica* **infestation?**

    Answer: *Clostridium spp*

29. **Pink eye in bovines is caused by**

    Answer: *Moraxella bovis*

30. **Calf hood vaccine is advisable for**

    Answer: Brucellosis

31. **Most susceptible species for Haemorrhagic septicemia is**

    Answer: Buffalo

32. **Erythritol sugar plays an important role in pathogenesis of**

    Answer: *Brucella spp*

33. **BCG is an attenuated form of**

    Answer: *Mycobacterium bovis*

34. **Coomb's test is employed for**

    Answer: Brucellosis and auto-hemolytic anaemia

35. **Microorganisms that can survive pasteurisation temperature are**

    Answer: Listeria and Coxiella

36. **Poll evil in horse is caused by**

    Answer: *Actinomyces bovis* and *Brucella abortus*

37. **Cell wall antigens of Corynebacterium are related to**

    Answer: Mycobacterium

38. **Calf diarrhoea is caused by**

    Answer: *Fusobacterium* sp./Bovine rota virus/Bovine viral diarrhea virus

39. **SMEDI disease in pigs is caused by**

    Answer: Porcine parvo virus

40. **The smallest virus is**

    Answer: FMD virus

41. **First virus studied in history**

    Answer: FMD virus

42. **In pox lesions which stage is involved in the spread of virus?**

    Answer: Vesicle

43. **Swollen head syndrome in poultry is caused by**

    Answer: Type A and B pneumoviruses

44. **'Negri bodies' for the diagnosis of rabies can be detected using**

    Answer: Seller's stain

45. **Which virus has distinctive wheel like appearance?**

    Answer: Rota virus

46. **Attenuation of virus was first introduced by**

    Answer: Louis Pasteur

47. **The reservoir host of rabies is**

    Answer: Vampire bats

48. **The first animal virus against which a genetically engineered vaccine was produced is**

    Answer: FMD virus

49. **Fowl typhoid is produced by**

    Answer: *Salmonella gallinarum*

Chapter 9

Veterinary Parasitology

1. **Corridore disease is caused by**

   Answer: *Theileria parva/lawrensi*

2. **Which is the most pathogenic fluke of poultry birds?**

   Answer: *Prosthogonimus ovatus*

3. **Which is known as Indian liver fluke?**

   Answer: *Fasciola gigantica*

4. **Billiaryamphistomiasis in swamp buffalo is caused by?**

   Answer: *Gigantocotyle explanatum*

5. **Gillar and pittoo is caused by**

   Answer: Immature amphistomiasis in Sheep and goat (Spread by *Indoplanorbis exustus*)

6. **Nasal granuloma/snoring disease is caused by**

   Answer: *Schistosoma nasale*

7. **Dhobi's itch/swimmer's itch/clam digger's itch is caused by**

   Answer: Non-human schistosomes and avian schistosomes

8. **Humpsore is caused by?**

   Answer: *Stephanofilaria asamensis*

12. **Which is known as 'Whip worm'?**

    Answer: Trichuris

13. **Anopheles acts as vector for**

    Answer: *Plasmodium spp,Dirofilaria immitis, Seratia digitata*

14. **Tabanus acts as a vector for**

    Answer: Anthrax, Surra and Equine infectious anemia virus

15. **Boiled rice like gravid segments in faeces of ruminants is due to tapeworm**

    Answer: *Moneizia sp*

16. **Gravid segments of which tapeworm in dog appear as cucumber seed?**

    Answer: *Dipylidium sp*

17. **The nematode that affects young poultry birds**

    Answer: *Ascaridia sp*

18. **Which lungworm has a higher prevalence in India?**

    Answer: *Dictyocaulus viviparus*

19. **Drug used for control of surra is**

    Answer: Quinapyrmine sulphate, Isometamidium chloride

20. **Winter coccidiosis in cattle is associated with**

    Answer: *Eimeria zuernii*

21. **The most pathogenic cooccidia in cattle is**

    Answer: *Eimeria zuernii*

22. **Which coocidial species affects goats?**

    Answer: *Eimeria arlongi*

23. **How to control parasite in field conditions?**

    Answer:

    - ☆ Herd sanitation: The herd should be cleaned in a regular frequency so that the manure is cleaned. The floor should be washed with lime at least once in a week to kill the parasite larvae and eggs.
    - ☆ Restriction in mixing of manure and feed: As manure contains egg of parasite so its mixing with feed should be restricted
    - ☆ Fecal sample examination: Periodical fecal sample examination should be conducted to identify the worm. Depending upon the test result the anthelminthic should be chosen.

- ✰ Mass deworming: Deworming should be carried out among the entire mass at a time to build herd immunity. Slow rotation between anthelminthics may be conducted to prevent the development of drug resistance. Always a full dose of deworming should be applied based on fecal sample test report, to control the worm load inside the body.
- ✰ Animal grouping: In order to properly treat the animals, groups of animals should be made based on how susceptible they are to parasites. Young animals, should be kept in a separate group because they are frequently more vulnerable than adult animals.
- ✰ Grazing management: Over grazing raises the risk of both ecto and endo parasite infestation. Strategy should be taken to control the over grazing also the field, which is reached in the infective stage of parasites, may be avoided. In hot and dry weather larvae die quickly, so the pasture should be exposed to sun light and heat so that the hay or pasture become worm free.
- ✰ Pasture rotation: Internal parasite eggs become infectious after six days from the date of passing through livestock manure. The field with overloaded parasitic larvae should be divided with temporary fencing for maintaining the pasture rotation. Animals should graze in a single land for six days and from the next day on another land.

24. Impact of parasites on health of animal and how to combat it?

Answer: Animal health and welfare can suffer from parasites in the following ways:

- ✰ Blood loss: As both internal and external parasites suck blood, it is substantial to cause anaemia and followed by death
- ✰ Diarrhoea: GI parasites cause profuse diarrhoea which may lead to death.
- ✰ Reduced appetite: All kind of parasites cause inappetence either directly or indirectly resulting in debilitation in animal health which make animals more susceptible to other diseases.
- ✰ Transmission of diseases: Many parasites act as vectors of various fatal diseases and which are transmitted from one sick animal to another healthy animal.
- ✰ Open sores: External parasites like house flies cause sore on open wound of skin of livestock.
- ✰ Grazing behaviour: Due to parasitic infestation the grazing behaviour of domestic animals are reduced.
- ✰ Reduced production: Due to parasitic infestation ultimately the side effect observed on production loss of farm animals which leads to economic loss to producers.

25. What are the common names of different worms

Answer:

NEMATODE

Parasite	*Common Name*	*Other Important Points*
Oesophagostomum sp.	Nodular worm	Black foetid diarrhoea/ pimply gut
Trichostrongylus colubriformis	Black scour or bankrupt worm	
Haemonchus contortus	Barber's pole worm/ stomach-worm/wireworm	most pathogenicBottle-jaw
Ostertagia ostertagi	Brown stomach worm/ Brown hair worm	morocco leather
Paramphistomum sp	Rumen fluke	-
Gongylonema verrucosum	Rumen gullet worm or gullet worm	-
Cooperia punctata	Cattle bankrupt worm	-
Ascaris suum	-	Milk spot
Toxascaris leonine/T. canis/T. cati	Arrow headed worm or Arrow worm	-
Family- Strongylidae	Palisade worm	-
Heterakis gallinarum	Caecal worm	-
Parasite	Common name	Other important points
Oxyuris equi	Pinworm of Horse/rectal worm	Rat-tailed
Enterobius vermicularis	Pinworm or seat worm of man	
Strongylus vulgaris		Verminous aneurysm
Stephanurus dentatus	Kidney-worm of pig	
Syngamus trachea	Gapeworm/forked worm	Gapes
Ancylostoma caninum	Hookworm of dog	
A.Tubaeforme	Hookworm of cat	
A.duodenale/N. americanus	Hookworm of man	
Bunostomum trigonocephalum	Hookworm of sheep and goats	Bottle-jaw
Globocephalus sp.	Hookworm of pig	
Dioctophyma renale	Giant kidney worm	
Bunostomum phlebostomum	Hookworm of cattle	

Parasite	*Common Name*	*Other Important Points*
Dictyocaulus filaria	Lungworm of sheep	
D.viviparus	Lungworm of cattle	Husk or hoose
Metastrongylus sp.	Lungworm of pigs	
Thelazia rhodesii	Eyeworm	
T.lachrymalis	Eyeworm of horse	
T. bubalis	Eyeworm of buffalo	
Dirofilaria immitis	Dog heartworm	
Setaria equine	Abdominal worm of equine	
S.digitata	Abdominal worm of cattle	
Stephanofilaria assamensis		Hump sore "Cascado"
Stephanofilaria zaheeri		Ear sore
Onchocerca volvulus		River blindness
Drancunculus medinensis	Guinea-worm	
Trichuris spp.	Whip-worm	

TREMATODE

Parasite	*Common Name*	*Other Important Points*
Dicrocoelium dendriticum	Lancet liver fluke	Slime balls
Clonorchis sinensis	Oriental or Chinese liver fluke	Cholangitis and cholangio hepatitis
Prosthogonimus ovatus	Oviduct fluke of poultry	Shell-less egg
Fasciola sp.	Liver fluke	Pipe-stem liver
Paragonimus westermanii	Lung fluke	
Paramphistomes	Rumen fluke or conical fluke	
Gigantocotyle explanatum	Disease condition called Biliary amphistomosis	
Family- Schistosomatidae	Blood fluke	Furcocercous cercariae
Schistosoma nasalis		Nasal schistosomasis" snoring disease" of cattle, goats and horses in India
S.hematobium		Urinary or vesicalschisto-somasis
S.indicum, S.spindale, S. incognitum		Hepato-intestinal schistoso-masis
Cercarial dermatitis is commonly known as 'swimmer's itch or 'dhobi's itch in India'clam-diggers' itch, 'hunters' itch, 'rice paddy' itch, lakeside disease'(Japan)		

CESTODES

Parasites	*Infective Stage*	*Common Name*	*Other Important Points*
Anoplocephala perfoliata	Cysticercoid in oribatid mite	Lappetted cestode	
Paranoplocephala mamillana	Cysticercoid in oribatid mite	Dwarf tapeworm of horse	
Thysanosoma actinioides		Fringed tapeworm	
Davainea proglottina	Cysticercoid in gastropod mollusks	Most pathogenic tapeworm of poultry	*Haemorrhagic enteritis*
Cotugnia diagnopora		Double-pored tapeworm of poultry	
Dipylidium caninum	Cysticercoids in fleas (Ctenocephalidescanis or c. felis or Pulexirritans) and doc louse (Trichodectiscanis)	Double-pored tapeworm of dog	
Hymenolepis nana	Direct life-cycle (important)	Dwarf tape worm of rodents,simian primates and man	
Taenia saginata	*Cysticercus bovis*		Measly beef
T. solium	*Cysticercus cellulosae*	Pork tapeworm	*Measly porkNeuro-cysticercosis or ocular cysticercosis in man*
T. ovis	*Cysticercous ovis*		
T. hydatigena	*Cysticercous tenuicollis* (mostly in sheep)		*Haemorrhagic and fibrotic tract in liver* (*Int. host*)
T.pisiformis	C. *pisiformis* (in Rabbit,hares and rodents)		
T. multiceps	*Coenurus cerebralis* (sheep,goat)		*Gid or Staggers*
T. serialis	*Coenurus serialis*		
Echonococcus granulosus	Hydatid cyst		*Unilocular hydatidosis*

Parasites	*Infective Stage*	*Common Name*	*Other Important Points*
E. multilocularis	Hydatid cyst		
Diphyllobothrium latum	1. Procercoid in body cavity of cyclops 2. Plerocercoid in fish	Broad fish tapeworm	*A macrocytic hypochromic anaemia develops resulting from a competition between parasite and host for vitamin* B_{12}

Chapter 10

Veterinary Pathology

1. **Saw dust liver in poultry carcasses is a typical necropsy finding in**

   Answer: Salmonellosis

2. **Pathological condition Noma is an example of**

   Answer: Acute gangrenous stomatitis or cancrum oris.

3. **White liver disease in sheep and goats occur due to deficiency of**

   Answer: Cobalt

4. **Shaggy heart appearance commonly associated with**

   Answer: Fibrinous Pericarditis

5. **Floating kidney is a common congenital anomaly observed in**

   Answer: Cat

6. **White spotted kidney in the calves are associated with**

   Answer: *Leptospira* sp.

7. **Etiology of enzootic hematuria in cattle occurs due to**

   Answer: Ingestion of Bracken fern

8. **Kumri in Horses is caused by**

   Answer: *Setaria digitata* (presence of larvae of *S. digitata* at C.N.S)

9. **Enzootic ataxia in new born lambs is attributed to**

   Answer: Copper deficiency and excess Molybdenum

10. **Common site for lodgement of uroliths in dog**

    Answer: Urinary bladder

11. **Hepatosis dietetica in pigs associated with a deficiency of**

    Answer: Selenium and Vit. E

12. **Pipe stem liver in necrosis associated with**

    Answer: Fascioliasis

13. **Bracken fern poisoning results in deficiency of**

    Answer: Thiamine

14. **Cold mastitis results due to**

    Answer: *Leptospira* sp.

15. **Pearly eye is a clinical feature associated with**

    Answer: Marek's Disease

16. **Almond shaped eye in poultry is a characteristic feature observed in**

    Answer: ILT

17. **Aetiology of 'Symptomatic anthrax' in cattle is**

    Answer: *Clostridium chauvoei*

18. **Watery whites of egg in poultry birds associated with outbreaks of**

    Answer: IB

19. **Typical 'Button Ulcer' in intestinal tract is observed in**

    Answer: Hog cholera

20. **Fatty liver and kidney syndrome in poultry results due to deficiency of**

    Answer: Biotin

21. **Type of Aflatoxin which is most toxic**

    Answer: AFB1

22. **Dropped jaw condition is met in**

    Answer: Rabies

23. **Etiology of Hjarre's disease in poultry birds**

    Answer: Avian pathogenic *E. coli*

24. **Malignant Jaundice in Dog is caused by**

    Answer: Babesiosis

25. **Typical horse hoof/nail head pattern of leison in poultry liver is characteristic**

    Answer: Black head disease caused by *Histomonas meleagridis*

26. **Black disease is in sheep is seen as a complication with**

    Answer: *Fasciola hepatica*

27. **Histamine is secreted by which cell?**

    Answer: Basophils

28. **The cell that acts as the first line of cellular defence is**

    Answer: Neutrophils

29. **Antibodies are produced from which cells?**

    Answer: Plasma cells

30. **Biphasic type of Vanden Berg reaction is observed in**

    Answer: Toxic Jaundice

31. **What is anthracosis?**

    Answer: Deposition of carbon particles in the lungs

32. **Eosinophils are the inflammatory cells mostly seen in what type of infection?**

    Answer: Parasitic infections

33. **When the suppurative inflammation involves the connective tissue diffusely, it is called**

    Answer: Cellulites

34. **Small focal suppurative area in the hair follicle or sebaceous gland is known as**

    Answer: Furuncle

35. **In tuberculosis, the type of giant cells seen is**

    Answer: Langhan's giant cell

36. **What type of necrosis seen in TB?**

    Answer: Caseation necrosis

37. "Bread and butter" pericarditis is an example of which inflammation?

Answer: Fibrinous inflammation

38. What type of inclusion body observed in canine distemper?

Answer: Cytoplasmic and Intranuclear inclusions

39. Which stain is used for the demonstration of Negri bodies?

Answer: Seller's stain

40. Define metaplasia

Answer: Transformation of one type of tissue into another is called metaplasia

41. What is Inflammation?

Answer: An inflammation is "The complicated biological reaction of vascular tissues to potentially detrimental stimuli, such as pathogens, damaged cells, or irritants."

42. What are the cordial signs of Inflammation?

Answer: An acute inflammation is characterized by

a) Rubor (redness)
b) Calor (heat)
c) Tumor (swelling)
d) Dolor (pain)
e) functio laesa (loss of function)

43. How cold application and warm application reduces the inflammation?

Answer: Cold application: In acute inflammation application of cold at 15 °C or less promotes Vaso-constriction and reduces the inflammatory exudate.

Warm application: Warm application at 40 to 45 °C is beneficial in severe inflammation which may leads to gangrene. It promotes the Vaso-dilation to restore blood supply.

44. Enlist the terminology of inflammations of different organs.

Answer:

Sl.No.	*Organ*	*Inflammation*	*Sl.No.*	*Organ*	*Inflammation*
1	Mouth (Buccal cavity)	Stomatitis	29	Cervix	Cervicitis
2	Tongue	Glossitis	30	Uterus	Metritis
3	Gum	Gingivitis	31	Endometrium	Endometritis
4	Pharynx	Pharyngitis	32	Oviduct	Salpingitis

Sl.No.	Organ	Inflammation	Sl.No.	Organ	Inflammation
5	Nasal mucous membrane	Rhinitis	33	Prepuce	Posthitis
6	Sinus	Sinusitis	34	Glans penis	Balanitis
7	Larynx	Laryngitis	35	Prepuce and Glans penis	Balanoposthitis
8	Trachea	Tracheitis	36	Testis	Orchitis
9	Bronchi	Bronchitis	37	Bone	Osteitis
10	Alveoli	Alveolitis	38	Cartilage	Costochondritis
11	Air sac	Airsacculitis	39	Bone, bone marrowand muscle	Osteomyelitis
12	Lungs	Pneumonia	40	Joints	Arthritis
13	Oesophagus	Oesophagitis	41	Synovial inflammation	Synovitis
14	Stomach	Gastritis	42	Meninges	Meningitis
15	Rumen	Rumenitis	43	Brain	Encephalitis
16	Abomasum	Abomasitis	44	Brain and Meninges	Maningoen-cephalitis
17	Proventriculus	Proventriculitis	45	Udder	Mastitis
18	Intestine	Enteritis	46	Conjuctiva	Conjunctivitis
19	Duodenum	Duodenitis	47	Cornea	Keratitis
20	Ileum	Ileitis	48	Ear	Otitis
21	Liver	Hepatitis	49	Muscle	Myositis
22	Gallbladder	Cholecystitis	50	Skin	Dermatitis
23	Pancreas	Pancreatitis	51	Endocardium	Endocarditis
24	Bile duct	Cholangitis	52	Pericardium	Pericarditis
25	Kidney	Nephritis	53	Myocardium	Myocarditis
26	Urinary bladder	Cystitis	54	Artery	Arteritis
27	Urethra	Urethritis	55	Vein	Phlebitis
28	Vagina	Vaginitis	56	Peritoneum	Peritonitis

45. What is necrosis? Classify necrosis.

Answer: Necrosis is the pathological death of a cell or group of cells in a living being.

- ☆ Coagulative necrosis: In hypoxic condition due to coagulation of protein necrosis occurs.
- ☆ Liquefactive necrosis: The tissue to change into a viscous liquid mass.

- ☆ Gangrenous necrosis: Necrosis caused due to formation of gangrene due to less blood supply to the tissue.
- ☆ Caseous necrosis: Can be considered a combination of coagulative and liquefactive necrosis typically caused by mycobacteria, fungi and some foreign substances.
- ☆ Fat necrosis: As a result of activated lipases' necrosis occurs on fatty tissues, including those of the pancreas.
- ☆ Fibrinoid necrosis: Caused due to immune-mediated vascular damage.

46. What is gangrene?

Answer: The death of a large region or mass of tissue due to a lack of blood supply, any disease or an injury is known as gangrene.

47. State the etiology and symptoms of gangrene.

Answer:

Etiology:

- ☆ Certain bacteria release huge toxin which leads to gangrene.
- ☆ Burn or frost bite
- ☆ Strong acid or alkali
- ☆ If nerve and blood supply is interfered by any trauma.
- ☆ Due to any obstruction gangrene may develop.

Symptoms:

a) Dry gangrene:

- ☆ Dead tissue loses volume and become dry.
- ☆ normal appearance of tissue is lost and color turns to black or brown.

b) Moist gangrene:

- ☆ Enlargement of the tissue due to accumulation of blood and other fluids.
- ☆ There will be severe pain.
- ☆ Color of tissue is changed to blackish to pinkish.
- ☆ Discharge may be observed with foul smell.

Chapter 11

Veterinary Public Health

1. **Small pox vaccine was developed by**

   Answer: Edward Jenner

2. **When is World Environmental day celebrated?**

   Answer: 5th June

3. **Epidemiological triad is an interaction of**

   Answer: Agent, host, environment

4. **Zoonoses day is celebrated on**

   Answer: July 5th

5. **Sweet curdling of milk is due to the species of**

   Answer: *Bacillus cereus*

6. **Immediate test to judge the quality of milk is**

   Answer: Organoleptic test

7. **Yeasty flavour in dairy products is due to**

   Answer: *Geotrichum candidum*

8. **Cold sterilization means**

   Answer: Flash pasteurization

9. **Well established protozoan disease transmitted through milk**

   Answer: Toxoplasmosis

10. **Rotten egg odour in water is due to**

    Answer: Algae

11. **The natural inhabitant of a bacteria in the udder is**

    Answer: *Staph aureus*

12. **Undulant fever is due to**

    Answer: *Brucella spp*

13. **Travellers diarrhoea is caused by**

    Answer: Bacteria mainly *E.coli*

14. **The emerging pathogen in milk**

    Answer: *Yersinia enterocolitica*

15. **Septic sore throat is due to**

    Answer: *Streptococcus pyogenes*

16. **Black colour of milk product is due to**

    Answer: *Pseudomonas nigrificans*

17. **The cold sterilization of milk can be done by**

    Answer: Lactoperoxidase system

18. **Specific germicidal substance in milk**

    Answer: Immunoglobulins

19. **Milk from Mastitis case**

    Answer: Has more alkailinity

20. **If milk is adulterated with water the boiling point of milk**

    Answer: Decreases

21. **The previous indicator organism for pasteurization**

    Answer: *Mycobacterium tuberculosis*

22. **LP system is related with**

    Answer: Germicidal property of milk

23. The term Zoonoses was coined by

Answer: Rudolf Virchow

24. Tuberculosis is

Answer: Direct zoonosis

25. In Japanese encephalitis infection pig acts as

Answer: Amplifier

26. Vector for dengue transmission is

Answer: *Aedes aegypti*

27. The causative agent of hydatidosis is

Answer: *Echinococcus granulosus*

28. Bilateral conjunctivitis in human is caused by which virus

Answer: New Castle disease virus

29. Boiling test on meat detects

Answer: Abnormal odour

30. Abattoir fever is the synonym of

Answer: Q fever

31. Enzootic abortion causing organism

Answer: *Campylobacter spp*

32. Sterne vaccine is used for the bacterial disease

Answer: Anthrax

33. Rice field worker's disease is the synonym of

Answer: Leptospirosis

34. Stuttgart disease in dogs is caused by

Answer: *Leptospira spp*

35. Which bacteria convert lactose into lactic acid?

Answer: *Staphyllococcus auerus*

36. Shipping fever causing organism

Answer: *Pasteurella multocida*

37. Black death causing organism

Answer: *Yersinia pestis*

38. How do milk borne infections take place?

Answer: Direct contact with diseased cows, contaminated tools or surfaces, poor hygiene habits, incorrect handling and storage, or intake of unpasteurized or raw milk may all result in milk-borne infections.

To prevent these infections, proper hygiene, cleaning and sanitization of equipment and surfaces, proper storage and handling, and pasteurization of milk are crucial.

Since milk contains so many different nutrients as a result germs, especially pathogens, flourish in it. Bacteria may grow and spread by using a variety of milk components. The metabolites that is produced by microbes include lactic and other organic acids, gases, enzymes, flavouring chemicals, colours, toxins, and other substances. The quality of milk may be impacted by these metabolites, which may be advantageous or detrimental. Due to the inherent hazards, it is advised, raw milk should never be consumed by anybody, at any time, for any reason.

39. Name a few diseases that are transmitted through milk?

Answer:

a) Tuberculosis - *Mycobacterium tuberculosis and Mycobacterium bovis*
b) Brucellosis or Malta fever – *Brucella abortus*
c) Diphtheria - *Corynebacterium diphtheriae*
d) Q Fever - *Coxiella burnetti*
e) Infectious hepatitis - Hepatitis A virus
f) Salmonellosis–*Salmonella spp.*
g) Enterobacteria – *E. coli*

40. What is zoonosis? Name different types of zoonotic diseases.

Answer: A zoonosis is an infectious disease that can spread from an animal to people. These diseases can be transmitted through direct contact with infected animals, consumption of contaminated food or water, or exposure to contaminated surface. Symptoms can range from mild to severe and potentially life–threating.

Sl.No.	*Group*	*Disease*	*Pathogens*	*Animals Involved*	*Mode of Transmission*
1	Viral Zoonosis	Bird flu or Avian Influenza	Influenza A virus subtype H5N1	Wild birds, domesticated birds such as chickens	Close contact
2		Rabies	Rabies virus	Commonly – dogs, bats, monkeys, foxes, cattle, goats, sheep, horses, mongooses, cats *etc.*	Through saliva by biting, or through scratches from an infected animal
3		Swine influenza	A new strain of the influenza virus endemic in pigs (excludes H1N1 swine flu, which is a human virus).	Pigs	Close contact
4		Ebola virus disease (Haemorrhagic fever)	Ebolavirus spp.	Chimpanzees, gorillas, orangutans, fruit bats, monkeys, shrews, forest antelope and porcupines	Through body fluids and organs
5		Hantavirus disease	Hantavirus spp.	Deer mice, cotton rats and other rodents	Exposure to feces, urine, saliva or bodily fluids
6		Hepatitis E	Hepatitis E virus	Domestic and wild animals	Contaminated food or water
7		Japanese encephalitis	Japanese encephalitis virus	Pigs, water birds	Mosquito bite
8		Kyasanur Forest disease	Kyasanur Forest disease virus	Rodents, shrews, bats, monkeys	Tick bite
9		Monkeypox	Monkeypox virus	Rodents, primates	Contact with infected rodents, primates, or contaminated materials
10		Nipah virus infection	Nipah virus (NiV)	Bats, pigs	Direct contact with infected bats, infected pigs

Sl.No.	*Group*	*Disease*	*Pathogens*	*Animals Involved*	*Mode of Transmission*
11	Viral Zoonosis	Orf	Orf virus	Goats, sheep	Close contact
12		Rift Valley fever	Phlebovirus	Livestock, buffaloes, camels	Mosquito bite, contact with bodily fluids, blood, tissues, breathing around butchered animals or raw milk
13		West Nile fever	Flavivirus	Birds, horses	Mosquito bite
14		Zika fever	Zika virus	Chimpanzees, gorillas, orangutans, monkeys, baboons	Mosquito bite, sexual intercourse, blood transfusion and sometimes monkey bites
15		Severe acute respiratory syndrome (SARS)	SARS coronavirus	Bats, civets	Close contact, respiratory droplets
16		COVID-19	Severe acute respiratory syndrome coronavirus 2	Suspected: bats, felines, raccoons dogs, minks. White-tailed deer	Suspected: bats, felines, raccoon dogs, minks. White-tailed deer
17	Bacterial Zoonosis	Anthrax	*Bacillus anthracis*	Commonly - grazing herbivores such as cattle, sheep, goats, camels, horses, and pigs	Ingestion, inhalation or skin contact of spores
18		Brucellosis	*Brucella* spp.	Cattle, goats, pigs, sheep	Contact with infected animals, fetal materials or animal products contaminated with the bacteria
19		Plague		*Yersinia pestis*	Rabbits, hares, rodents, ferrets, goats, sheep, camels

Sl.No.	*Group*	*Disease*	*Pathogens*	*Animals Involved*	*Mode of Transmission*
20		Chlamydiosis/ Enzootic abortion	*Chlamydophila abortus*	Domestic livestock, particularly sheep	Close contact with postpartum ewes
21		Tuberculosis	*Mycobacterium bovis*	Infected cattle, deer, llamas, pigs, domestic cats, wild carnivores	Milk, exhaled air, sputum, urine, faeces and pus from infected animals
22	Bacterial Zoonosis	Foodborne illnesses (Commonly diarrheal diseases)	*Campylobacter spp., Escherichia coli, Salmonella spp., Listeria spp., Shigella spp., Trichinella spp.*	Animals domesticated for food production (cattle, poultry)	Raw or undercooked food made from animals and unwashed vegetables contaminated with feces
23		Leptospirosis	*Leptospira interrogans*	Rats, mice, pigs, horses, goats, sheep, cattle, buffaloes, opossums, raccoons, mongooses, foxes, dogs	Direct or indirect contact with urine of infected animals
24		Psittacosis	*Chlamydophila psittaci*	Pigeons, sparrows, ducks, hens, gulls and many other bird species	Contact with bird droplets
25	Rickettsial Zoonosis	Q fever	*Coxiella burnetii*	Livestock and other domestic animals such as dogs and cats	Inhalation of spores, contact with bodily fluid or faeces
26		Rocky Mountain spotted fever	*Rickettsia rickettsii*	Dogs, rodents	Tick bite
27	Protozoal Zoonosis	African sleeping sickness	*Trypanosoma brucei rhodesiense*	Range of wild animals and domestic livestock	Transmitted by the bite of the tsetse fly
28		Chagas disease	*Trypanosoma cruzi*	Armadillos, Triatominae (kissing bug)	Contact of mucosae or wounds with feces of kissing bugs.
29		Giardiasis	*Giardia lamblia*	Beavers, other rodents, raccoons, deer, cattle, goats, sheep, dogs, cats	Ingesting spores and cysts in food and water contaminated with feces

Sl.No.	*Group*	*Disease*	*Pathogens*	*Animals Involved*	*Mode of Transmission*
30		Leishmaniasis	*Leishmania* spp	Dogs, rodents, other animals	Sand fly bite
31		Toxoplasmosis	*Toxoplasma gondii*	Cats, livestock, poultry	Exposure to cat feces, contaminated soil, water, grass, unwashed vegetables *etc.*
32	Parasitic Zoonosis	Cysticercosis and Taeniasis	*Taenia solium, Taenia saginata*	Commonly – pigs and cattle	Consuming water, soil or food contaminated with the tapeworm eggs (cysticercosis) or raw or undercooked pork contaminated with the Cysticerci (Taeniasis)
33		Toxocariasis	*Toxocara* spp.	Dogs, foxes, cats	Ingestion of eggs in soil, fresh or unwashed vegetables or undercooked meat
34	Parasitic Zoonosis	Trichinosis	*Trichinella* spp.	Rodents, pigs, horses, bears, walruses, dogs, foxes, crocodiles, birds	Eating undercooked meat
35		Fasciolopsiasis	*Fasciolopsis buski*	Pigs	Eating raw vegetables such as water spinach
36	Prion Zoonosis	Bovine spongiform encephalopathy	Prions	Cattle	Eating infected meat

41. Name some meat borne diseases?

Answer:

Bacteria: *Campylobacteriosis, Salmonellosis, Listeriosis, Pathogenic Escherichia coli (E. coli), Yersiniosis*

Bacterial toxins: Toxins of *Staphylococcus aureus, Clostridium perfringens, Clostridium botulinum* and *Bacillus cereus*

Viruses: Calicivirus (including norovirus), Rotavirus, Hepatitis A virus, Hepatitis E virus

Parasites: *Trichinellosis, Toxoplasmosis, Cryptosporidium, Giardiosis*

42. Define the following: Pandemic, panzootic, endemic, epidemic, epizootic, reverse zoonosis

a) Pandemic: An infectious disease that is prevalent throughout a whole nation or the world at one particular time is called pandemic disease.

b) Panzootic: A panzootic is an animal disease outbreak that affects an extensive region, such as an entire nation, continent, or even the entire world. A pandemic is the term used for its human population equivalent.

c) Endemic: When an infection is consistently present or maintained at a baseline level in a particular population or populated area without additional infections being introduced into the group as a result of travel or other similar means, the infection is said to be endemic in that population or area.

d) Epidemic: An epidemic is when a disease spreads quickly through a population, infecting a large number of hosts in a short amount of time.

e) Epizootic: Similar to an epidemic in humans, an epizootic is a disease outbreak in a population of nonhuman animals over a large area.

f) Reverse zoonosis: Reverse zoonosis, also referred to as zooanthroponosis or anthroponosis, is the term used to describe a pathogen reservoir in humans that can spread to non-human animals.

43. State the relationship among outbreak, epizootic and panzootic.

Answer: An "outbreak" of an epizootic disease may happen in a particular area, an "epizootic" may happen in a larger area, and a "panzootic" may occur when it spreads widely.

Chapter 12

Animal Genetics and Breeding

1. Name different breeds of cattle

Sl.No.	*Breed Name*	*Home Tract*	*Purpose*
Indigenous Breeds of cattle			
1.	Sahiwal	Montgomory dist. Of Pakistan	Milch Breed
2.	Gir	Gir forest, Gujarat	Milch Breed
3.	Red sindhi	Sindh province in Pakistan	Milch Breed
4.	Deoni	AP, Karnataka, Maharastra	Milch Breed
5.	Tharparkar	Ajmer, Jodhpur Dist of Rajasthan	Milch Breed
6.	Rathi	Rajasthan	Dual Breed
7.	Hariana	Rohtak, Hissar, Karnal	Dual Breed
8.	Mewati	UP, Rajasthan	Dual Breed
9.	Kankrej	Katch and Ahmedabad, Gujarat	Dual Breed
10.	Ongole	Ongole, Nellore Dist of AP	Dual Breed
11.	Gaolao	MP, AP	Dual Breed
12.	Krishna valley	AP, Karnataka	Dual Breed
13.	Dangi	Ahmednagar, Gujarat	Dual Breed
14.	Nagori	Rajasthan	Draught Breed
15.	Malvi	Malva region of MP	Draught Breed
16.	Kherigarh	Kheri Dist of UP	Draught Breed
17.	Kenketha	Banda Dist. of UP	Draught Breed

Sl.No.	Breed Name	Home Tract	Purpose
18.	Nimari	Nimar and Indore, MP	Draught Breed
19.	Panwar	UP	Draught Breed
20.	Bachaur	Bhagalpur, Bihar	Draught Breed
21.	Khillari	Sholarpur, Satatra Dist of MS	Draught Breed
22.	Amritmahal	Mysore, Karnataka	Draught Breed
23.	Hallikar	Tumkur, Mysore dist. Of Karnataka	Draught Breed
24.	Bargur	Coimbatore, Tamil Nadu	Draught Breed
25.	Kangyam	Coimbatore, Tamil Nadu	Draught Breed
26.	Siri	Sikkim, Darjeeling	Draught Breed
27.	Red kandhari	Maharastra	Draught Breed
Exotic Breeds			
28.	Holstein Friesian	Netherland	Milch Breed
29.	Brown Swiss	Switzerland	Milch Breed
30.	Jersey	Jersey Island	Milch Breed
31.	Ayrshire	Ayrshire country, Scottland	Milch Breed
32.	Guernsey	Gurensey	Milch Breed
33.	Hereeford	England	Milch Breed
34.	Angus	Scottland	Milch Breed
Crossbred Developed in India			
35.	Taylor	Patna, Bihar	Shorthorn and Jersey with local cows
36.	Jersind	Allahbad, UP	Jersey x Red Sindhi
37.	Sunandini	Kerala	Brown Swiss x Non descript
38.	Frieswal	Merrut, UP	3/8 to 5/8 Friesian x Sahiwal
39.	Karan Fries	NDRI, Karnar (Haryana)	Friesian x Tharparkar
40.	Karan Swiss	NDRI, Karnar (Haryana)	Brown Swiss x Sahiwal
41.	Jerthar	Bangalore, Karnataka	Jersey x Tharparkar

2. Name some buffalo breeds found in India

Sl.No.	Breed Name	Home Tract	Purpose
1	Murrah	Haryana, Punjab	Milch Breed
2	Nilli Ravi	Ferozpur, Punjab	Milch Breed
3	Surti	Surat, Kaira Dist. of Gujarat	Milch Breed
4	Mehsana	Gujarat	Milch Breed
5	Jafrabadi	Gujarat	Milch Breed

3. Name some breeds of pig

Sl.No.	Breed Name	Home Tract
Exotic Breeds		
1	Large White Yorkshire	Yorkshire, England
2	Middle White Yorkshire	Yorkshire, England
3	Berkshire	Berkshire
4	Landrace	Denmark
5	Tamworth	Central England
6	Duroc	United States
7	Chester White	USA
Indigenous Breed		
1	Doom	Assam
2	Purnea	Bihar and Jharkhand
3	Mali	Tripura
4	Ghurrah	Uttar Pradesh
5	Ghoongroo	West Bengal

4. Name some important indigenous and exotic goat breeds

Sl.No.	Breed Name		Home Tract	Purpose
1	North Temperate Region	Gaddi	Himachal and UP	Fibre
2		Chanthangi	Ladakh	Fibre
3		Chegu	Himachal and UP	Fibre
4	North Western Arid and Semi Arid	Sirohi	Rajasthan, Gujarat	Meat
5		Marwari	Rajasthan, Gujarat	FIbre
6		Beetal	Punjab, Haryana	Dairy, Meat
7		Barbari	UP, Rajasthan	Dairy, Meat
8		Jamunapari	UP	Dairy, Meat
9		Surti	Gujarat	Dairy, Meat
10	Southern Penninsular	Sangamneri	Maharastra	Meat
11		Osmanabadi	Maharastra	Meat
12		Malabari	Keralla	Meat
13	Eastern Region	Ganjam	Orissa	Meat
14		Black Bengal	West Bengal	Meat
15	**Exotic Breeds**	Alpine	Alps	Milk Production
16		Anglo Nubian	UK	Milk and Meat
17		Toggenberg	Toggenberg	Skin
18		Saanen	Switzerland	Milk

5. Name some breeds of rabbit.

Sl.No.	*Breed Name*	*Home Tract*	*Purpose*
1	Indian Hare or black naped hare	Indian subcontinent, Java	Pelt
2	Angora Rabbit	Angora, Turkey	Fur (woolly)
3	Soviet Chinchilla	USSR	Fur and Meat
4	Newzealand White	US	Meat and fur
5	Grey Giant	USSR	Fur and Meat
6	Californian white	California	Meat and fur
7	White Giant	Earstwhile Soviet Union	Fur and Meat

6. Name some sheep breed found in India

Sl.No.	*Breed Name*		*Home Tract*	*Purpose*
1	North Temperate Region	Bhakarwal	Jammu and Kashmir	Carpet Wool
2		Chanthangi	Ladakh	Carpet Wool
3		Gurej	Gurej (Kashmir)	Carpet Wool
4		Karnah	Karnah (Kashmir)	Apparel Wool
5		Kashmir	Kasmir Valley	Apparel Wool
6	North Western Arid and Semi Arid	Muzzafarnagri	Western UP	Meat, Carpet Wool
7		Jalauni	UP	Meat, Carpet Wool
8		Munjal	Punjab, Haryana	Meat, Carpet Wool
9		Hisardale	Hissar	Apparel Wool
10		Chokla	Rajasthan	Meat, Carpet Wool
11		Jaisalmeri	Jodhpur	Meat, Carpet Wool
12	Southern Penninsular	Deccani	Maharastra	Meat, Carpet Wool
13		Bellari	Karnataka	Meat, Carpet Wool
14		Mechari	Tamil Nadu	Meat, Carpet Wool
15		Hasan	Karnataka	Meat
16		Nilgiri	Tamil Nadu	Apparel Wool
17	Eastern Region	Balangir	Orrisa	Meat, Carpet Wool
18		Ganjam	Orrisa	Meat, Carpet Wool
19		Garole	West Bengal	Meat
20		Bonpala	Sikkim	Meat, Carpet Wool
21	**Exotic Breeds**	Merino	Spain	Fine Wool
22		Rambouillet	France	Fine Wool
23		Hampsire	Scottland	Medium Wool
24		Lincoin	England	Long Coarse Wool

Sl.No.	*Breed Name*		*Home Tract*	*Purpose*
25	Crossbred Developed in India	Avivastra	Avikanagar	Chokla/Nali + Ramboulliet/Merino
26		Hissardale	GLF, Hissar	Bikaneri + Australian Merino
27		Kashmir Merino		Gaddi/Bhakarwal + Ramboulliet/Merino
28		Avikalin	Avikanagar	Malpura + Ramboulliet

7. Name some poultry breed found in India

Sl.No.	*Breed Name*		*Home Tract*	*Purpose*
1	Indian Native Breeds	Aseel	Chattisgarh, Orissa, AP	Show, Cock Fight
2		Chittagong/Malay	Meghalaya, Tripura	Dual Purpose
3		Kadaknath	MP	Meat
4		Busra	Gujarat, Maharastra	Broiler
5		Haringhata Black	West Bengal	Dual Purpose
6		Nicobari	Andaman and Nicobar	Dual Purpose
7		Kalasthi	AP	Dual Purpose
8		Miri	Assam	Dual Purpose
9		Mewari	Rajasthan	Dual Purpose
10	Crossbreds from different research institutes	Jharsim	Birsa Agriculture University, Ranchi	Dual Purpose
11		Kamrupa	Developed in Assam Agriculture University	Dual Purpose
12		Pratapdhan	MPUAT, Udaipur	Dual Purpose
13		CARI NIRBHEEK	Developed in CARI, Izatnagar (Aseel Cross)	Backyard farming
14		CARI SHYAMA/ Kalamashi	Developed in CARI, Izatnagar (Kadaknathl Cross)	Meat
15		CARI Sonali	Developed in CARI, Izatnagar	Layer
16		CARIBRO Dhanraja	Developed in CARI, Izatnagar	Broiler
17		Gramapriya	Developed in ICAR, Hyderabad	Layer
18		Sindhi	Developed in ICAR, Hyderabad	Dual Purpose

Sl.No.	Breed Name		Home Tract	Purpose
19		Vanaraja	Developed in ICAR, Hyderabad	Backyard farming
20		Swarnadhara	Developed in KVAFSU, Bidar	Layer
21	Quails	CARI Uttam	Developed in CARI, Izatnagar	Dual Purpose
22		CARI Pearl	Developed in CARI, Izatnagar	Dual Purpose
23		CARI Ujjawal	Developed in CARI, Izatnagar	Dual Purpose
24	Guniea Fowl	Kadambari	Developed in CARI, Izatnagar	Dual Purpose
25		Chitambari	Developed in CARI, Izatnagar	Dual Purpose
26		Swetambari	Developed in CARI, Izatnagar	Dual Purpose
27	Turkey variety	CARI Virat	Developed in CARI, Izatnagar	Broiler

8. **Which is the heaviest breed of cattle in India and its breeding tract?**

   Answer: Kankrej and its breeding tract is Gujarat and Rajasthan.

9. **Cattle breed from West Bengal and Sikkim**

   Answer: Siri

10. **Name a Cross bred cattle developed in IVRI, Bareilly**

    Answer: Vrindavani

11. **Peculiar Sai chal or $1^{1}/_{4}$ paces of gait in observed in which breed**

    Answer: Kankrej

12. **Prominent fore head and Long pendulous ears folded like a leaf are characteristics of which breed?**

    Answer: Gir

13. **Name a Cross bred cattle developed in NDRI, Karnal**

    Answer: Karan Swiss, Karan Fries

14. **Name some milch breeds of Indian origin**

    Answer: Gir, Shaiwal, Red Sindhi, Tharparkar

15. Name some dual purpose breeds of Indian cattle

Answer: Hariana, Ongole, Kankrej, Deoni, Dangi

16. Name some draught purpose breeds of Indian cattle

Answer: Hallikar, Amritmahal, Kangyam, Siri

17. Castrated male cattle is called as

Answer: Steer

18. Sound produced by cattle or buffalo is called

Answer: Bellowing

19. What is wallowing

Answer: Rolling or floundering in mud or in water by riverine or swamp buffalo. Buffaloes apparently wallow for two reasons to regulate body temperature and to control parasites. Swine also wallow.

20. Mozzarella cheese is made from which milk

Answer: Buffalo milk

21. During dehorning which nerve is blocked by local anaesthesia?

Answer: Cornual nerve block

22. In pig which identification method is commonly used?

Answer: Ear notching

23. During checking of dentition of heifer, you observed two incisor, two pre-molar and three molars, so what will be the age of that heifer?

Answer: 2-2.5 years

24. Normal body temperature of cattle

Answer: 101.8-102.4°F

25. Joria wool is obtained from

Answer: Kathiawari sheep breed

26. Tallest goat breed of India

Answer: Jamunapari

27. What is the largest and heaviest sheep breed in India?

Answer: Muzaffarnagari

28. Mention one pig breed from West Bengal

Answer: Ghoongroo

29. The process to induce donor for shedding several ova at a time is called

Answer: Super ovulation

30. Full form of MOET

Answer: Multiple Ovulation Embryo Transfer

31. When two purebred animals of different breed is mated, it is called

Answer: Crossbreeding

32. Improvement of biological quality in hybrid offspring is known as

Answer: Heterosis

33. In which type of pedigree evaluation parents are chosen on the basis of phenotype performance?

Answer: Progeny Testing

34. What is gummer condition of sheep?

Answer: Beyond six years of age, sheep gradually losses their teeth due to ageing. When a sheep losses all of its incisor teeth, it is called a gummer.

35. Pashmina is obtained from which goat breed?

Answer: Chegu and Chanthangi

36. Fine wool has 10 per cent medulation, is it true or false?

Answer: False. Fine wool has no medullation.

37. When a gene located in locus influences effect of other gene at another locus is called

Answer: Epistasis

38. When mating is done between a crossbred animal and one of its pure parent is called

Answer: Back crossing

39. Hallikar cattle breed originated from which state

Answer: Karnataka

40. Name some goat breeds from Western Arid and semi arid areas of India

Answer: Jamunapari, Barbari, Beetal, Surti *etc.*

41. Name some pig breeds of India

Answer: Ghoongroo, Niang Megha, Tenyi Vo, Doom

42. Name some Eastern region sheep breed of India

Answer: Chottanagpuri, Ganjam, Bonpala, Garole

43. Panch Kalyani (Nili Ravi) buffalo breed originated from

Answer: Punjab

44. What is the smallest cattle breed in India?

Answer: Vechur from Kerala

45. National Bureau of Animal Genetic Center is situated in

Answer: Karnal, Haryana

46. Central Institute for research on goats is situated in

Answer: Mathura, Uttar Pradesh

47. National Research Center on yak is situated in

Answer: Dirang, Arunachal Pradesh

48. National Research Center on Pig is situated in

Answer: Rani, Guwahati

49. National Research Center on camel is situated in

Answer: Bikaner, Rajasthan

50. Central sheep and wool research Institute is situated in

Answer: Avikanagar, Rajasthan

51. Ram from which sheep breed is used for fighting

Answer: Katchaikatty black

52. Best dairy goat of south east Asia is

Answer: Jamunapari

53. Milk queen of goat world is which breed of goat?

Answer: Saanen (Switzerland)

54. In a layer farm HDEP is calculated 80 per cent per year. What does it mean? Is it desirable?

Answer: NO. Average HDEP should be more than 85 per cent. It means the egg production in that farm is low.

55. The potential capacity of the female to produce functional ova is termed as

Answer: Fecundity

56. The pressure inside the artificial vagina for collecting semen should be

Answer: 45-55 mm HG

57. Sudden variations resulting from chemical structural or positional changes of genes is called

Answer: Gene mutation

58. The fraction of the superiority of parents transmitted to their offspring is called

Answer: Heretability

59. Project directorate on Foot and Mouth Disease is situated at

Answer: Mukteswar, Uttarakhand

60. What is the native track of Black Bengal goat? What are the breed characteristics of the Black Bengal goat?

Answer: The breed is widely distributed throughout West Bengal and adjoining parts of the neighbouring states, *viz.*, Bihar, Jharkhand, Orissa, Assam and parts of Tripura. The breed is equally prevalent in Bangladesh. But the main home tract of the breed is throughout West Bengal.

Breed Characteristics:

Body: It is a small-legged goat, the shoulder and hips are of equal height. The female body looks triangular from the side, with a heavier posterior region. This character is less prominent in males.

Head profile: Majority of the animals possess straight head, followed by convex and concave type.

Beard: Bengal goats are also found to have beard in few cases particularly in old ages

Body hair:Generally hair coat of the breed is thin, smooth and shiny as required for higher heat tolerance.

Coat colour: Bengal goat possesses both pure and mixed coat colours. Pure colours are black, white, brown and grey. Mixed colours are formed by the combination of any two of the pure colours. Prevalence of black coat colour is maximum and for this reason the breed is often misnomer as "Black Bengal".

Ear: Ears are either erect or pendulous. However up to 10 cm in length, ears are mostly erect types. When length is more than 10 cm, relative proportion of pendulous type increases.

Horn: Two types of horn, *viz.*, curved and straight are found in Bengal goat.

Birth weight: 1.235 Kg ± 0.006 Kg

Slaughter age and weight: Optimum age of slaughter is 12 months with a slaughter weight of 12 Kg.

Litter size: 2 kidding in 14 months with 2 to 3 offspring.

61. What are the different sheep breeds available in West Bengal?

Answer: Sundarban area: Garole

North Bengal: Bonpala

Bankura-Purulia-West Bardhaman Districts: Chottonagpuri

East and West Midnapore: Ganjam

62. What is the native track of Garole sheep? What are the breed characteristics of Garole sheep?

Answer: The habitat of the Bengal breed of sheep known as Garole is Sunderbans (Southern part of West Bengal) comprising of 13 blocks of South 24-Parganas and 6 blocks of North 24-Parganas district.

Characteristics:

General conditions: Garole has a compact and square body with a small head, medium ears and a short thin tail. The fleece cover on the coat is not dense but covers almost the whole body and the greater part of the legs. Males are usually horned and females are polled.

Coat colour: Garole sheep have a light brownish coat colour. Very few sheep with completely black or white coat colour or black/white spot on the body can also be found.

Slaughter weight: It is a small sized animal with a relatively low body weight in comparison to medium and heavy breeds of sheep. The average adult body weight in males and females being 14.43 and 14.14 kg, respectively.

Birth weight: Average 0.82±0.03 Kg

Reproduction and breeding: maximum lambing takes place between December to February and August to September. The age at first service is 7 to 9 months and age at first lambing is 12 to 14 months. The average number of lambs born per ewe was 1.68.

63. What is the native track of Bonpala sheep? State the breed characteristics of Bonpala sheep?

Answer: The Bonpala breed is native to southern Sikkim and some parts of Nort Bengal.

Characteristics:

Coat colour: Fleece colour ranges from complete white to complete black with a number of intermediary tones.

General conditions: The animals are tall, leggy and well built. Ears are small and tubular. Both sexes are horned. Tail is thin and short. Fleece is coarse hairy and open. Belly and legs are devoid of wool.

Slaughter weight: Rams and ewes achieves about 15-20 kg weight during maturity.

64. State the characteristics of the Chottonagpuri and Ganjam breeds of sheep.

Answer: Chottonagpuri

Coat colour: Predominantly white and the rest are brown, grey and black. Undercoat white/grey; yields warm delicate fiber - pashmina (cashmere, pashm).

General conditions: Body and legs are small, have strong body and powerful legs. Ears are small, pricked and pointed outwards. Horns are large turning outward, upward and inward forming a semicircular ring.

Birth weight: Average birth weight is 2.1 kg.

Slaughter weight: Average live weight of buck is 20 Kg and doe is 20 kg

Reproduction and breeding: Kidding is once a year, normally single; Average age at first kidding is 20 months.

Ganjam

The Ganjam breed of sheep is native to the Ganjam, Koraput, Phulbani and parts of the Puri districts of Odisha.

Coat colour: Coat colour ranging from brown to dark tan, some have white spots on the face and body.

General conditions: Ears are of medium size and drooping. These are medium sized animals Nose line is lightly convex. Tail is medium long and thin. Males are horned but females polled. Fleece is hairy and short which is not shorn.

65. What is the native track of Ghungroo pig? State the breed characteristics of Ghungroo pig?

Answer: Ghungroo is an indigenous breed of pig first reported from North Bengal. It is popular among the local people because of high prolificacy and ability to sustain in low input system. This breed/strain produces high quality pork utilizing agricultural byproducts and kitchen wastes.

Characteristics:

Coat colour and general conditions: Ghungroo pigs are mostly black coloured, long tail, upwardly curved snout, large heart-shaped ears, with folded skin on face and neck, long and cylindrical barrel belly with a typical Bulldog face.

Reproduction and breeding: Litter size is 6-12 piglets, individually weigh about 1.0 kg at birth and 7.0 – 10.0 kg at weaning. The female pigs attain sexual maturity at 10 months and in males as early as 8 months.

Slaughter weight: The adult body is weighing about 55 to 60 kg.

66. In Animal Husbandry what does the word 'litter' means?

Answer: The word 'Litter' denotes

a) A group of young animals born to a single mother at the same time time

b) Various materials that are used for bedding, like sawdust, wood shavings, and feathers mixed with animal excreta are called litter.

67. What is breeding?

Answer: Breeding is a form of sexual reproduction that results in offspring. It is possible only between a male and a female animal or plant.

68. What is inbreeding?

Answer: When individuals or other organisms who are genetically closely related, mate or breed for production of offspring, it is referred to as inbreeding. Eg. Female common fruit flies choose mating with siblings over other males.

69. What is cross breeding?

Answer: Crossbreeding is the act of mating two purebred individuals who are from different breeds, variations, or even species in order to produce offspring. This is commonly practiced by breeders, especially when the desired traits would be beneficial to the offspring. Eg. Crossing of nondescript breed (*Bos indicus*) with exotic Jersey or Holstein Friesian breed (*Bos taurus*).

70. What is grading up?

Answer: Grading up is the mating of animals from two distinct breeds in which the animals of a native breed or genetic group are mated for multiple generations with an improved pure breed in order to acquire the superior characteristics of the superior recognized breed. Eg. Grading up of nondescript breed with superior Sahiwal or Gir breed.

71. What is Sire index?

Answer: The sire index is a measurement of a bull's heritability for milk output or any other attribute. The sire index or bull index is a mathematical measure of the sire's capability to transfer production ability.

72. For superior quality of wool what should be desired staple length?

Answer: Staple length >75mm is taken as superior wool

73. In which type of breeding offspring will be more homozygous?

Answer: Inbreeding

Chapter 13

Pharmacology

1. **What is MIC and MBC?**

Answer: The minimum inhibitory concentration (MIC) is a way of determining how sensitive a bacterium is to the antibiotic. *Pasteurella* species are very sensitive to the fluoroquinolones, as are Gram-negative bacilli (*e.g. E. coli*) and Gram-positive cocci (*Staphylococcus* spp.) as they have a low MIC.

Enterococci, Bordetella bronchiseptica and particularly *Streptococci* have the highest MIC and are therefore usually classified as resistant.

The minimum bactericidal concentration (MBC) is another interesting pharmacodynamic parameter. For bactericidal drugs it can be anticipated that MIC and MBC should be similar, while it is generally accepted that for bacteriostatic drugs MBC will be several times higher than MIC. Fluoroquinolones kill bacteria most rapidly when their concentrations are considerably above the MIC of the targeted micro-organism. Enrofloxacin should not be given to growing animals as cartilage damage has been reported as a potential side effect.

2. **What is bactericidal and bacteriostatic antibiotics? Give some examples.**

Answer:

☆ Bactericidal: The antimicrobials which kill the bacteria.

- Fluoroquinolones (*e.g.* Enrofl oxacin)
- β-lactam antibiotics (*e.g.* Penicillin)
- Aminoglycosides (*e.g.* Gentamicin)

- ☆ Bacteriostatic: The antimicrobials which inhibit the growth and multiplication of bacteria.
  - Sulphonamides (*e.g.* Sulfasalazine)
  - Tetracyclines (*e.g.* Oxytetracycline)
  - Chloramphenicol
  - Macrolides (Erythromycin)

3. What are the major features of Fluoroquinolones ?

Answer:

- ☆ Broad-spectrum bactericidal activity that includes Gram-negative and Gram-positive aerobic bacteria and mycoplasms.
- ☆ They are not active against anaerobes
- ☆ They should not be used as first-choice antibiotics in order to prevent the development of resistance
- ☆ The fluoroquinolones in veterinary use include:
  - ❖ Enrofloxacin
  - ❖ Ciprofloxacin
  - ❖ Marbofloxacin
  - ❖ Orbifloxacin
  - ❖ Difloxacin
  - ❖ Ibafloxacin

4. State the mechanism of action of β-lactam antibiotics.

Answer: The bactericidal effects are mediated by preventing bacterial cell wall synthesis and disrupting bacterial cell wall integrity. β-lactams bind to a series of enzymes involved in the final stages of cell wall synthesis. This leads to the formation of defective cell walls that are osmotically unstable and cell death usually results from lysis.

5. What is the main cause of penicillin degradation?

Answer: Hydrolysis is the main cause of penicillin degradation and can take place in the syringe when penicillin is mixed with another drug.

6. Why Sodium or Potassium salts of penicillins are used?

Answer: Sodium or potassium penicillin salts are suspended in an inert oil for prolong absorption of penicillin from the site of injection for 18 hours

7. What is depot penicillin?

Answer: Incorporation of the poorly soluble procaine penicillin in oil, prolongs absorption for 24 hours or more. Benzathine penicillin G is a repository salt of penicillin and absorption may be prolonged for 7 days or more. This is called depot penicillin.

8. State the Pharmacokinetics of Penicillin.

Answer:

- ☆ The physical and chemical properties, especially solubility, of penicillins are related to the structure of the acyl side chain and the cations used to form salts.
- ☆ High concentrations of these drugs are achieved in kidneys, liver and lung.
- ☆ Penicillins do not penetrate the CNS unless there is inflammation present.
- ☆ Metabolites are inactive and are excreted in the urine.

9. Classify Cephalosporins with examples.

Answer: There are total five generations of cephalosporines based. The successive generations are less absorbed orally, increased stability to gram negative β-lactamase and increased activities against gram negative bacteria.

- ☆ First generation: Cefazolin, Cefadroxil, Cefapirin, Cefaloridine *etc.*
- ☆ Second generation: Cefuroxime, Cefaclor *etc.*
- ☆ Third generation: Ceftriaxone, Cefotaxime, Ceftiofur, Ceftazidime, Cefoperazone, Cefixime, Cefpodoxime, Ceftizoxime *etc.*
- ☆ Fourth generation: Cefquinome, Cefepime ect.
- ☆ Fifth generation: Ceftobiprole, Ceftaroline

10. Name some β-lactamase inhibitors and why they are called as Suicidal antibiotics?

Answer: The agents which bind with the β-lactamase enzyme produced by gram positive and gram-negative bacteria. Examples: Clavulanic acid, Sulbactam and Tazobactam.

As these agents itself get degraded after binding to β-lactamase enzyme and protect other β-lactam antibiotics. So, these are called as suicidal antibiotics.

11. What are the major features of Aminoglycosides?

Answer:

- ☆ These are produced from strains of *Streptomyces spp.* and other bacteria.
- ☆ They have excellent water, but poor lipid, solubility and are thermodynamically stable over a wide range of pH values and temperatures.
- ☆ They are potentially nephrotoxic when given systemically and ototoxic due to binding to proximal tubules and inhibition of mitochondrial function.

- ☆ They function by irreversibly binding to bacterial ribosomes and interfering with mRNA translation.
- ☆ Gentamicin, streptomycin and neomycin are the most widely used agents in this group.

12. Give examples of Aminoglycoside antibiotics.

Answer: Streptomycin, Gentamicin, Neomycin, Kanamycin, Tobramycin, Amikacin *etc.*

13. What is the mechanism of action of Sulfonamides?

Answer: Sulfonamides compete with PABA and inhibits the production of bacterial folic acid.

14. What are the side effects of Sulfonamides?

Answer: Adverse drug reactions should be suspected in any dog that develops new clinical signs. Members of the sulfonamide group of antibiotics in particular have been implicated as a cause of adverse drug reactions in the dog with one survey reporting 82 per cent of antibiotic reactions being due to sulfonamides. Other findings include a 4 per cent incidence of lameness with their use and a predisposition for Dobermanns to be affected due to a difference in the metabolism of the drug compared with other breeds.

Sulfonamide shows type III hypersensitivity reaction causing signs such as sterile polyarthritis, blood disorders such as anaemia, neutropenia and thrombocytopaenia.

15. What is potentiated Sulfonamide?

Answer: The combination with other antimicrobial drugs (most commonly trimethoprim) reduces the minimum inhibitory concentration needed of both drugs and therefore reduces side effects. The combination of Sulfonamide group of drugs with Trimethoprim is called potentiated Sulfonamides.

e.g. Co-trimoxazole – combination of Sulfamethaxole and Trimethoprim.

16. Give some examples of tetracycline group of antibiotics.

Answer: Tetracycline, Chlortetracycline, Oxytetracycline, the synthetic drug Doxycycline *etc.*

17. State the mechanism of action of tetracycline group of antibiotics.

Answer: The antimicrobial activity of the tetracyclines is produced by binding to the 30S ribosomes of susceptible organisms and interfering with bacterial protein synthesis in growing or multiplying organisms.

18. Why tetracycline should be avoided just after parturition?

Answer: Ttracyclines have the ability to bind polyvalent cations like Ca++ and Mg++, which are crucial for several hormonal and enzymatic processes. Chelation of calcium can cause a severe lack of calcium in the blood, which results in hypocalcemia.

19. What are the characteristics features of Macrolide antibiotics? Give few examples.

Answer:

a) They are weak bases that are poorly absorbed.

b) Inhibit protein synthesis by binding to the ribosome.

c) They are mainly effective against Gram-positive organisms.

d) They are bacteriostatic at therapeutic concentrations, but can be slowly bactericidal, especially against *Streptococci*.

e) The antimicrobial action of erythromycin is enhanced by a high pH, with the optimum antibacterial effect at a pH of 8. Therefore, in an acidic environment, such as in an abscess, necrotic tissue or urine, the antibacterial activity is suppressed.

Example: Erythromycin, Tylosin, Azithromycin Tilmicosin

20. What are the characteristics features of of Lincosamides? Give examples.

Answer:

a) Used primarily to treat Gram-positive infections where there is resistance or intolerance to penicillins.

b) Inhibit protein synthesis by binding to the ribosome.

c) They penetrate bone well and are indicated in osteomyelitis and peridontitis.

d) Toxic in small mammals, where they can trigger a clostridial overgrowth.

e) There are two agents in this group: 1. Lincomycin 2. Clindamycin.

21. Describe about some major antifungal drugs

Answer:

A. Griseofulvin:

☆ Griseofulvin is a systemic antifungal agent effective against the common dermatophytes. It works by distorting the hyphae of the fungus and hence is fungi static rather than fungicidal. Its absorption from the gut is variable and is enhanced by high-fat meals and propylene glycol because of its low water solubility.

- ☆ Griseofulvin is contraindicated in pregnant animals because it is teratogenic; otherwise, it has good selective toxicity as it is preferentially taken up by susceptible fungi rather than by mammalian cells.
- ☆ Method of action – disrupts the mitotic spindle by interacting with the microtubules, stopping mitosis in metaphase.
- ☆ Metabolism – mainly in the liver at a rate approximately 6 times faster in dogs than in humans, which is the reason why the dose rate is much higher.

B. *Amphotericin B:*

- ☆ This agent is a polyene fungicidal antibiotic used to treat serious systemic mycoses, fungal septicaemia or fungal urinary tract infections. It is also a useful treatment for leishmaniasis.
- ☆ Amphotericin is highly plasma protein bound and penetrates into body fluids and tissues relatively poorly. It acts by binding to sterols in cell membranes, thereby impairing cell membrane permeability – this allows the leakage of cell electrolytes, resulting in cell death.
- ☆ The chemical structure of the drug is of a large macrolide lactose ring, one side of which is hydrophobic and the other side is hydrophilic, resulting in an amphipathic molecule.
- ☆ Once diluted in water, the drug is present in three forms: as soluble monomers (the active drug), soluble oligomers and insoluble aggregates (this last form is the most toxic).
- ☆ Amphotericin B is known for its nephrotoxicity, due to renal vasoconstriction, direct tubular damage and reduced glomerular filtration rate.
- ☆ One way to reduce its toxicity is to encapsulate the drug in liposomes or to dilute it in a solution of soya bean oil.

C. *Azole antifungal drugs – imidazoles and triazoles:*

- ☆ These are broad-spectrum antifungals including: Clotrimazole, miconazole, ketoconazole, fluconazole, itraconazole, enilconazole.
- ☆ Mode of action – inhibit synthesis of primary steroid of the fungal cell membrane, ergosterol. They are fungistatic at therapeutic doses. Ketoconazole is highly protein bound (> 98 per cent) and therefore does not penetrate into the CSF, seminal or ocular fluid to a significant degree but does enter mother's milk.
- ☆ It is metabolized in the liver and excreted in the bile.
- ☆ It is only soluble in acid aqueous environments (pH < 3) and therefore antacids decrease oral absorption.
- ☆ The main adverse effects are nausea and vomiting.

- ☆ Drug interactions are common because ketoconazole inhibits metabolism of other drugs due to being an inhibitor of cytochrome P-450.

22. Classify antiviral drugs used in veterinary medicine

Answer: The antivirals are the best grouped depending on which stage in viral replication they have their action.

i. ***Transcription***

- ☆ Idoxuridine and trifluridine: Incorporate themselves into viral and mammalian DNA strands, making them more susceptible to breakage. They are used topically in herpes keratitis.

  These drugs competitively inhibit the DNA polymerase but have side effects including gastrointestinal, neurological and haematological toxicities.

- ☆ Ribavirin: Purine analogue that inhibits a wide range of RNA and DNA viruses and its strongest activity is against RNA respiratory viruses (influenza A and B).

  It has several sites of action including inhibiting synthesis of guanine nucleotides. It can be given orally, i.v. and by aerosol - which produces the best results with the minimum side effects.

- ☆ Acyclovir (Zovirax) and Ganciclovir: The mode of action is to selectively inhibit the viral DNA polymerase and to incorporate themselves into the viral DNA strands causing termination of elongation. Effective against herpes virus.

  Acyclovir has a good selective toxicity and a high therapeutic index and is available as a topical, oral and i.v. preparation. It is minimally metabolized with > 70 per cent excreted in the urine.

- ☆ Zidovudine (AZT): It is thymidine analogue which is phosphorylated by cellular enzymes and then inhibit viral reverse transcriptase (an enzyme important in the replication of DNA) 100× more than it inhibits the mammalian enzyme, therefore making the drug selective in its actions and ensuring a low mammalian toxicity. Extensively used to control HIV infection.

  It has been used in cats to treat feline immune deficiency virus (FIV), an incurable disease that is spread mainly through bites.

  The host remains asymptomatic for months to years before secondary infections cause illness.

ii. ***Assembly***

- ☆ Amantadine and rimantidine: Water-soluble cyclic amines with antiviral activity against a narrow range of RNA viruses, including influenza A. They inhibit late-stage assembly of the virus.

23. What is anthelmintic drug?

Answer: Anthelmintics are a class of antiparasitic medications that kill or expel internal parasites and worms by which they can be eliminated from the body without causing significant damage to the host. They reduce the accumulation of harmful worm eggs or larva on the pasture as well.

24. What is the difference between vermicides and vermifuges?

Answer: Vermicides: When Anthelmintic kill the parasitic worms are called vermicides.

Vermifuges: When Anthelmintic remove the parasitic worms from GI tract by temporarily paralysing them they are called vermifuges.

25. What is broad spectrum anthelmintic?

Answer: When both mature and immature parasites, including larvae, are susceptible to the anthelmintic drugs those anthelminthic drugs are called as broad spectrum anthelminthic.

26. What should be the feature of a good anthelmintic drug?

Answer: The ideal anthelmintic -

a) should have broad spectrum of activity
b) should be easy to administer to a large number of animals
c) should have a wide margin of safety
d) should not require long withdrawal periods
e) should not cause any unpleasant side effects
f) should be economical to farmers.

27. Classify different types of anthelminthic drugs mostly used in Veterinary field.

Answer: Anthelmintics may be classified based on the effectiveness against different types of helminths into three broad groups:

A. Antinematodal drugs:

a) Benzimidazoles: Albendazole, Fenbendazole, Mebendazole, Oxibendazole, Oxfendazole, Triclabendazole *etc.* and Pro-benzimidazoles like Febental, Netobimin, Thiophanate
b) Macrocyclic lactones/Antibiotics: Ivermectin, Doramectin, Eprinomectin, Abamectin *etc.*
c) Imidazothiazoles: Tetramisole, Levamisole and Butamisole
d) Tetrahydropyrimidines: Pyrantel, and Oxantel
e) Piperazines: Piperazine and diethylcarbamazine
f) Substituted phenols and salicylanilides: Closantel

B. Anticestodal drugs:

a) Isoquinolones: Praziquantel and Epsiprantel

b) Salicylanilides: Niclosamide

c) Substituted phenols: Dichlorophen, Nitroscanate

d) Benzimidazoles: Albendazole, Fenbendazole, Mebendazole, Oxibendazole, Oxfendazole

C. Antitrematodal drugs:

a) Substituted phenols: Nitroxinil, Hexachlorophene, Bithionol

b) Salicylanilides: Cosantel, Rafoxanide, Oxyclozanide, Niclosamide

c) Aromatic amides: Diamfenetide

d) Sulphonamides: Clorsulon

e) Halogenated hydrocarbons: Carbon tetrachloride, Hexacloroethane

f) Isoquinolones: Praziquantel

g) Benzimidazoles: Albendazole, Fenbendazole, Triclabendazole

28. Mention some commonly used medicines act against ectoparasite and endoparasite both.

Answer: Closantel, Ivermectin, Doramectin

29. Mention the doses of commonly used anthelmintics in veterinary medicine.

Answer: Nematodes – Albendazole, Fenbendazole, Ivermectin, Doramectin, Piperazine

Medicine Group	*Drug*	*Dose*		
		Cattle and Buffalo	*Sheep and Goat*	*Dog*
Antinematodal	Albendazole	7.5 -10 mg/kg PO	10 mg/kg PO	25-50 mg/kg PO
	Fenbendazole	7.5 mg/kg PO	5 mg/kg PO	50 mg/kg PO
	Ivermectin	0.2 mg/kg SC	0.2 mg/kg SC	0.2-0.3 mg/kg SC
	Doramectin	0.2 mg/kg SC	0.2 mg/kg SC	0.2 mg/kg SC
	Levamisole	7.5 mg/kg SC or PO	7.5 mg/kg SC or PO	5-8 mg/kg PO
	Piperazine	110 mg/kg PO	110 mg/kg PO	80-120 mg/kg PO
Anticestodal	Praziquantel	-	10-15 mg/kg PO	5 mg/kg PO
	Niclosamide	50 mg/kg PO	100 mg/kg PO	100-150 mg/kg PO

Medicine Group	*Drug*	*Dose*		
		Cattle and Buffalo	*Sheep and Goat*	*Dog*
Antitre-matodal	Cosantel	5 mg/kg SC	10 mg/kg PO	-
	Rafoxanide	7.5 mg/kg PO	7.5 mg/kg PO	-
	Oxyclozanide	10-15 mg/kg PO	10-15 mg/kg PO	-

30. Mention some commonly used medicines act against ectoparasite.

Answer:

Medicine	*Group*
Amitraz	Tri-azeidentadiene
Cypermethrin	Pyrethroid
Deltametrin	Pyrethroid
Flumethrin	Synthetic pyrethroid
Permethrin	Synthetic pyrethroid
Propoxur	Carbamate

Chapter 14

General Questions

1. **What are the ARD schemes are going on at the field level at present in West Bengal?**

   - ☆ Chick Distribution Scheme: Input: Ten number of 28 days old chicks for each beneficiary. Training, Vaccination cost, Monitoring cost provided.
   - ☆ Goat Distribution Scheme: Per SHG Input: (10 female (Doe) with insurance, Medicine,i.e Dewormer, feed supplement, min mix, Monitoring and training cost provided.
   - ☆ Pig Distribution Scheme: Input: Each block will select 5 beneficiaries as cluster. Each of them will receive 2 females (Sow) except one will receive one sow and one boar, with insurance, Initial Feed cost, Medicine Dewormer, feed supplement, min mix, Monitoring and training cost, Existing Shed repairing cost provided.
   - ☆ Heifer Rearing scheme: Input: (1 heifer of 1 y age Body wt. Cross Bred: 70-80kg, Sahiwal/Gir: 70-90kg/per beneficiary with insurance, Initial Feed cost, Monitoring and training cost, Existing Shed repairing cost
   - ☆ MGNREGA convergence scheme: Target beneficiary: SHG group, shed cost will be provided by MGNREGA Input: Either 50 chicks or 50 ducklings.
   - ☆ Organization Animal Health Cum Awareness Camp:
   - ☆ Matir Srishti Project: Government of West Bengal has launched the "MatirSristi" Project in six Paschimanchal district with a view to transform barren land(Those plots are not used for agriculture due to low fertility) into green vegetation and to create all possible livelihood opportunities by dovetailing inputs from various line department/Schemes/Programmes

of Central and State Govt. for better agricultural output, Animal husbandry and Fisheries. ARD plays an important role for sustainable income generation to the poorer through different departmental schemes

- ☆ Assistance to Goat Farmers to strengthen Rural Micro-Level Goat Husbandry units in West Bengal. With the view to reduce mortality, improve fertility and growth of the existing goat, making practice of selling goat on the basis of body weight to increase return, to develop a greater number of goat husbandry based FPCs in future, the scheme was launched. To implement the scheme, cluster to be formed with 50 number of Goat farmers. Each farmer must have minimum 3 no. of does. Farmers will be provided with medicine for their goat, vaccination, training, health care monitoring *etc.* throughout the year for 2 years.
- ☆ FPOs and FPC: FPO: Farmers producer organization are group of rural producers coming together based on the principle of membership, to purse specific common interests of their members and developing technical and economic activities that benefit their members and maintain relations with partners operating in their economic and institutional environment.

Objectives of FPO:

i. To provide holistic and broad-based supportive ecosystem

ii. To enhance productivity through efficient, cost-effective and sustainable resource use and realize higher returns through better liquidity and market linkages.

iii. To provide effective capacity building to FPOs to develop agriculture/ animal husbandry entrepreneurship skills to become economically viable and self-sustaining.

iv. To provide handling and support to new FPOs upto 5 years from the years of creation in all aspects of management of FPO, inputs, production, processing and value addition, market linkage, credit linkage and use of technology *etc.*

The services provided by Farmer's Producer's organization:

i. Marketing services (input supply, output marketing and processing market information.

ii. Financial services (savings, loans, and other forms of credit)

iii. Technology services.

iv. Education services (business skills, health, nutrition)

v. Welfare services *etc.*

FPCs: Farmer's Producer's Companies: A producer company is basically a body, corporate registered as producer company under companies act,1956 and shall carry on or relate to any of following activities.

i. Production, harvesting, processing, procurement, grading, handling, marketing, selling export of primary produce of the members or import of goods or services for their benefit.

ii. Rendering technical services, consultancy services, training education, research and development and all other activities for the promotion of the interests of its members.

iii. Generation transmission and distribution of power, revitalization of land and water resources, their use, conservation and communication relatable to primary produce

- ✰ Fodder, Minikit distribution Scheme: Selected fodder seed or cutting is distributed among beneficiaries.
- ✰ KCC-AH: As per specific guideline animal owner may apply for bank loan for recurring expenditure of animal (i.e feeding *etc.*) under the guidance of block ARD officials.

2. **How many BAHC, ABAHC, SAHC, Polyclinic have been established under ARD dept. in the West Bengal?**

   Answer: BAHC: 342, ABAHC: 273, SAHC: 102, Polyclinic + MDVH: 8+2

3. **What is the recommendation of ICMR (Indian council of Medical Research) for per capita,milk, egg and meat requirement and what is the availability in West Bengal vis-a vis India?**

   Answer:

Food	ICMR Recommended/ per capita	Availability in West Bengal/per capita	Availability in India/per capita
Milk	280 gm/per capita/per day	179 gm/per capita/per day	444 gm/per capita/per day
Meat	34 gm/per capita/per day	19.5 gm/per capita/per day	18.68gm/per capita/per day
Egg	182 egg/per capita/per year	117 egg/per capita/per year	95 egg/per capita/per year

4. **What are the chemicals used to preserve the animal carcass body and what the term used to mention this chemicals mixture?**

   Answer: This chemical is collectively known as Embalming Chemicals which is composed of Formaldehyde, Glutaraldehyde, Methanol and other solvents.

5. **What are the Vaccination programme is going on at field level at present?**

Answer: FMDCP, PPRCP, Brucella CP and LSDCP

6. **What are the different vaccines produced at IAH and VB, Kolkata?**

Answer: Vaccines produced at IAH and VB. Kolkata

Sl.No.	*Name of the Vaccine*	*Type of the Vaccine*	*Doses*	*Route of Inoculation*
1	Anthrax Spore vaccine	Live attenuated	100	S/C
2	Black Quarter vaccine	Inactivated adjuvanated	20	S/C
3	HS vaccine	Inactivated adjuvanated	20	S/C
4	Goat Pox vaccine	Live freeze dried (Cell culture)	100	S/C
5	PPR vaccine	Live freeze dried (Cell culture)	100	S/C
6	Swine fever	Live freeze dried (lapinized)	5	S/C
7	Fowl Cholera vaccine	Inactivated adjuvanated	100	S/C
8	Ranikhet Disease (F strain)	Live freeze dried	100	I/N or I/O
9	Ranikhet Disease (R2B strain)	Live freeze dried	200	I/M
10	Fowl Pox (PPCEVL)	Live freeze dried	100	Feather follicle or I/M
11	Fowl Pox (CEVL)	Live freeze dried	100	Feather follicle or I/M
12	Duck Cholera vaccine	Inactivated adjuvanated	100	I/M
13	Duck Plague	Live freeze dried	50	I/M

7. **What should we do as Veterinary Officer at field level or what are the duties of a Veterinary Officer**

Answer: Firstly, we should gather few basic information of the particular block such as the animal population in the area, the prevalent disease, fodder cultivation and locally available low-cost feed ingredient *etc.* The following duties to be performed as Veterinary Officer:

A. Attend health centers, treat the cases, advice animal owners in respect of health care management system.

B. Attend all outbreaks in respective jurisdiction and take all possible effort to combat epidemic.

C. Arrange mass inoculation and undertake parasitic control camps.

D. Visit, supervise the functions of all institutions under his/her control.

E. Arrange health cams in all G.P.s periodically.

F. Perform A.I. and responsible for proper scientific programme in the respective jurisdiction.

G. Maintain all registers and office records and inspect those of the sub-centres.

H. Assist BLDO in successful implementation of all schemes.

I. Examine pathological samples collected from ailing animals and sending them to nearby pathology cum diagnostic laboratory.

J. Submit activity report of his dispensary and of the units under his/her control to the BLDO.

K. Training of farmers on animal husbandry programmes.

8. **Name the domestic ruminant with highest BMR.**

Answer: Goat

9. **Tell the life Span of RBC of animal and chicken.**

Answer: Avg 100 days, Chicken. 28-35 days

10. **Normal temperature of different animal**

Answer: Cattle: 100-102.5°F

Buffalo. 99-102°F

Goat. 101.5-103.5°F

Fowl. 105.8-107.6°F

Horse: 99-100.5°F

11. **What is the cattle population in India?**

Answer: According to 20th Livestock census (2019) it is 192.49 million

12. **What is the Indian position in cattle population in world?**

Answer: 2nd in the world

13. **Which state has the largest cattle population in India?**

Answer: West Bengal

14. **What is the buffalo population in India?**

Answer: 109 million (2019 census)

15. **What is the Indian position in Buffalo population in world?**

Answer: 1st in the world

16. How much does the agricultural sector contribute in the total GDP of India?

Answer: 17.9 per cent (2021-22)

17. How much does the Livestock sector contribute tothe GDP of India?

Answer: 4.6 per cent (2021-22)

18. Which product contributes most to the livestock GDP?

Answer: Milk contributes the most part (More than 70 per cent). Followed by meat, dung and egg

19. What is unique practice for goat feeding?

Answer: Tethering

20. What are the average life span and maximum recorded life span of cattle and goat?

Answer: Cattle: Avg 20-25 years, maximum recorded 30yrs

Goat: Avg 10-15 years, maximum recorded 18 years.

21. Licking/Gnawing (vice) is caused due to deficiency of

Answer: Minerals.

22. Quarantine period of how many days covers almost all diseases?

Answer: 1 Month.

23. Pigs are mostly identified by

Answer: Ear Notching.

24. Shortest gestation period is seen in

Answer: Bitch.

25. Which is used as calf-hood vaccine?

Answer: Brucellosis.

26. Most common cause for heavy neonatal mortality in calves is due to

Answer: Calf scour.

27. White meat is commonly obtained from

Answer: Pig and Poultry.

28. Mention the name of the leading State in India for Livestock Production as per 20th Livestock Census or Livestock Production Statistics-2020

Answer:

Sl.No.	*Feature*	*Name of the State*
1	Highest poultry population	Tamil Nadu
2	Largest duck population	West Bengal
3	Highest cow milk production	Tamil Nadu.
4	Highest buffalo milk production	Uttar Pradesh
5	Highest goat milk production	Rajasthan
6	Highest goat meat production	West Bengal
7	Highest Poultry meat production	Haryana
8	Highest exotic/crossbred cattle population	Tamil Nadu
9	Highest cattle population	West Bengal
10	Highest pig population	Assam
11	Highest livestock population	Uttar Pradesh
12	Highest Buffalo population	Uttar Pradesh
13	Highest goat population	Rajasthan
14	Highest sheep population	Telengana
15	Highest Pig meat production	Bihar
16	Highest Sheep meat production	Telangana

29. Hemoglobin content in various domestic animals ranges

Answer: 8-16 gm/dl

30. Holdup of milk is caused by

Answer: Adrenalin.

31. For the production of 1liter of milk, how much blood passes through udder?

Answer: 400-500 ltr

32. Which is called milk vein?

Answer: Subcutaneous abdominal vein

33. Which amino acid is predominant in cow milk?

Answer: Isoleucine.

34. India's first 100 per cent organic state is

Answer: Sikkim

35. Mention the position of India for livestock production and population in the world as per the 20th Livestock Census

Sl.No.	Feature	Position of India in World
1	Livestock Population	1st
2	Cattle Population	2nd
3	Buffalo Population	1st
4	Sheep Population	3rd
5	Goat Population	2nd
6.	Poultry population	6th

36. What is the total milk production of India?

Answer:221.06 MMT per year (Basic Animal Husbandry Statistics(Govt. of India)-2022)

37. What is the total milk production of West Bengal?

Answer: 6.414 MMT per year (Basic Animal Husbandry Statistics(Govt. of India)-2022)

38. State the position of India in world vis-a vis highest position of a state in India in respect of milk, meat and egg production and per capita availability.

Answer:

Item	Milk Production	Meat Production	Egg Production	Wool Production
Position of India in world	1st	8th	3rd	9th
Highest producing state in India	Rajasthan (15.05 per cent)	Maharashtra (12.25 per cent)	Andhra Pradesh (20.41 per cent)	Rajasthan (45.91 per cent)

Source: Basic Animal Husbandry Statistics (Govt. of India)-2022.

Per Capita availability

Item	Milk	Meat	Egg
State with highest per capita availability in India	Punjab (1271 gm)	Telengana (22.79 kg/annum)	Andhra Pradesh (450 egg)

Source: Basic Animal Husbandry Statistics (Govt. of India)-2022.

39. What will be your suggestions to the beneficiaries regarding rearing, vaccination *etc.* of distributed Chicks/Ducklings under Govt. scheme in field level.

Answer:

a) Supplied chicks should be kept in a close confinement to protect them from adverse weather condition or predators.

b) Saline water or glucose water should be supplied

c) If any chick exhibits any disease symptoms those should be separated from the fit ones and treated accordingly.

d) Contact with respective Pranimitra or Pranisebi of concerned GP, for vaccines under the supervision of Veterinary officer of the concerned block

e) 28 days old chicks are supplied under chick distribution programme. At the brooding unit all the chicks are vaccinated against Marek's Disease on the 1st day and Ranikhet disease (F1 strain) on the 7th day. After distribution within 3-4 days, Ranikhet disease (F1 Strain) vaccine is given. After 30-45 days (8th week to 10th week of age) Ranikhet disease (R2B strain) is administered which can be again repeated between 16th-18th weeks of age. Fowl pox (PPCEVL) freeze dried live vaccine can be given 6th-7th week of age onwards and Fowl-pox (CEVL) freeze dried live vaccine can be administered 14th weeks of age.

40. The silver revolution is associated with an increase in the production of

Answer: Eggs

41. Kadaknath is a breed of poultry from

Answer: Madhya Pradesh

42. How much energy can be produced from one egg?

Answer: 90 Kcal

43. Built up litter provides vitamins like

Answer: Animal protein factor (Vit B12) and Riboflavin (Vit B2)

44. What is the brooding space per young chick ?

Answer: 6 sq inch

45. What is the egg laying age of Layer pullet?

Answer: 20 weeks

46. What are the dentition formula of different animal?

Answer: **Cattle/Buffalo/Sheep/Goat**

I: C: PM: M (Upper/Lower)::

0/8: 0/0 :6/6 : 6/6

Total 32

Pig

I: C: PM: M (Upper/Lower)::

6/6: 2/2 : 8/8 : 6/6

Total 44

47. Mention floor space requirements of different animal in housing system.

Answer:

i. Adult cattle – 50 sq ft
ii. Calf- 15-20 sq ft
iii. Buffalo- 25-35 sq ft
iv. Sheep and Goat- 5-10 sq ft
v. Pig- 10-15 sq ft
vi. Broiler – 1 sq ft
vii. Layer – 3 sq ft

48. Blood spot in egg of poultry marks

Answer: Low level of Vitamin A

49. Phosvitin is a protein present mainly in

Answer: Egg yolk

50. Avidin complexes with

Answer: Biotin

51. The vitamin absent in chicken egg is

Answer: Vitamin C

52. Mushy/soft chick is due to

Answer: Un-sanitary incubator conditions

53. Ducks are very susceptible to deficiency of

Answer: Niacin

54. Typical arched backward position of duck is a characteristic of

Answer: Duck plague

55. Mention the name of different Milk Unions in West Bengal.

Answer:

Sl.No.	*Name of Milk Unions*	*District*
1	Bhagirathi Milk Union	Murshidabad
2	Kisan Milk Union	Nadia
3	Midnapore Milk Union	Paschim Medinipur
4	Damodar Milk Union	Hooghly
5	Bardhaman Milk Union	Purba Bardhaman
6	Ichhamati Milk Union	North 24 Parganas
7	Sundarban Milk Union	South 24 Parganas
8	Mayurakshi Milk Union	Birbhum
9	Kansabati Milk Union	Bankura
10	Howrah Milk Union	Howrah
11	Manbhum Cooperative Milk Producers Union Ltd.	Purulia
12	Tamralipta Milk Union	Purba Medinipur

Species-wise Livestock Population in West Bengal as per 20th Livestock Census

District	*Cattle*	*Buffalo*	*Sheep*	*Goat*	*Pig*
Alipurduar	520443	2209	7476	281764	58991
Coochbehar	1226670	6397	63824	486974	7372
Darjeeling	203881	6992	969	164834	57166
Kalimpong	48915	129	82	64109	13208
Jalpaiguri	727592	5381	8169	512322	36680
Uttar Dinajpur	1091590	12384	1521	885282	25809
Dakshin Dinajpur	532056	1920	6295	598137	41055
Maldah	1038763	38439	32919	1376487	70969
Murshidabad	1199817	66783	51415	1751276	8236
Nadia	816780	17157	24669	924339	4923
North 24 Paraganas	697601	34443	34356	780001	7241
South 24 Paraganas	1019495	11709	82258	791587	7348
Kolkata	1003	459	93	3625	335
Howrah	226388	5724	237	157017	362
Hooghly	912745	35229	1655	886410	16671
Purba Bardhaman	1532669	58942	135965	1370985	21327
Paschim Bardhaman	273637	22682	6498	256143	16635
Birbhum	1185333	94938	159206	1168796	38374

District	*Cattle*	*Buffalo*	*Sheep*	*Goat*	*Pig*
Bankura	1491831	64427	71889	1064468	20648
Purulia	915274	77650	186925	966681	30510
Purba Medinipur	1093499	263	5948	475230	1891
Paschim Medinipur	1758443	37649	18172	872869	25438
Jhargram	563491	29015	52345	440004	29167
Grand Total	**19077916**	**630921**	**952886**	**16279340**	**540356**

Source: 20th Livestock Census report.

Species-wise Livestock Population in Indian States and UT as per 20th Livestock Census

Sl. No.	State/UT	Total Exotic Cattle (Male+ Female)	Total Indigenous Cattle (Male + Female)	Total Cattle (Male + Female)	Total Buffalo (Male + Female)	Total Sheep (Male + Female)	Total Goat (Male + Female)	Total Pig (Male + Female)
1	A and N Islands	14260	20919	35179	3700	5	64761	40488
2	Andhra Pradesh	2239885	2337858	4577743	6219499	17626971	5522133	91958
3	Arunachal Pradesh	6462	332234	338696	6379	7345	159740	271463
4	Assam	712974	10140290	10853264	421715	332100	4315173	2099000
5	Bihar	4013660	11297513	15311173	7719794	213377	12821216	343434
6	Chandigarh	8940	4438	13378	12177	0	998	138
7	Chhattisgarh	257895	9716929	9974824	1174722	180229	4005657	526901
8	D and N Haveli	1165	38566	39731	997	84	7548	0
9	Daman and Diu	224	1596	1820	374	68	987	0
10	Delhi	60987	25446	45671	162142	278	30470	76346
11	Goa	27502	32718	60220	27207	662	9446	35480
12	Gujarat	3384417	6226448	9610865	10543250	1787263	4867744	658
13	Haryana	870989	949541	1820530	4368023	288370	334640	108240
14	Himachal Pradesh	1067211	759082	1826293	646565	791345	1108413	2477
15	Jammu and Kashmir	1436602	1096013	2532615	690829	3247503	1730218	1215
16	Jharkhand	591911	10596859	11188770	1350313	641183	9121173	1276973
17	Karnataka	3898075	4560842	8458917	2984560	11050728	6169392	323836
18	Kerala	1249821	82692	1332513	101504	1482	1359161	103863

Sl. No.	State/UT	Total Exotic Cattle (Male+ Female)	Total Indigenous Cattle (Male + Female)	Total Cattle (Male + Female)	Total Buffalo (Male + Female)	Total Sheep (Male + Female)	Total Goat (Male + Female)	Total Pig (Male + Female)
19	Lakshadweep	1158	1297	2455	16	0	43188	0
20	Madhya Pradesh	1679338	17055853	18735191	10307131	324585	11064524	164616
21	Maharashtra	4540352	9384574	13924926	5603692	2680329	10604883	161000
22	Manipur	17663	206546	224209	36230	5921	38697	235255
23	Meghalaya	31860	870165	902025	15714	15679	397503	706364
24	Mizoram	19682	24246	43928	2109	485	14820	292465
25	Nagaland	16970	59895	76865	15654	361	31602	404695
26	Odisha	1553347	8323590	9876937	458324	1279149	6393452	135162
27	Puducherry	66067	5745	71812	2395	2445	73630	880
28	Punjab	2047458	425873	2473331	4015947	85560	347949	52961
29	Rajasthan	2297860	11614597	13912457	13693316	7903857	20840203	154808
30	Sikkim	115748	31160	146908	1144	2016	90506	27320
31	Tamil Nadu	7675558	1793941	9469499	518795	4500491	9888746	66772
32	Telangana	596260	3621726	4217986	4226306	19063058	4934673	177992
33	Tripura	114248	610194	724442	7131	5460	360204	206035
34	Uttar Pradesh	5892293	12897013	18789306	33016785	984725	14480025	408678
35	Uttarakhand	571316	1275303	1846619	866318	284615	1371971	17659
36	West Bengal	3336735	15684764	19021499	630921	952886	16279340	540356

Source: 20th Livestock Census report.

www.ingramcontent.com/pod-product-compliance
Ingram Content Group UK Ltd.
Pitfield, Milton Keynes, MK11 3LW, UK
UKHW020220041026
15470UKWH00012B/729